THERAPEUTIC EFFECT ON DYSFUNCTION IN PANCREAS

By :

Sarmishta Srikantam

ACKNOWLEDGEMENT

Here is a small effort to extend my gratitude to each and every one who travelled with me all along the journey of my Ph.D degree programme.

I firstly thank **God**, who gave all the strength physically and mentally, to complete the chosen path without any compromise. I thank the Department of Biochemistry, Bharathi Women's College, Chennai for being a safest place to work, with good ambience and laboratory infrastructure.

At this juncture, I would like to express my deepest thanks to my research supervisor, **Dr. A. Geetha**, M.Sc., M.Phil., Ph.D., who had faith in me while accepting me, as a research student under her supervision. She was at the peak of her career with loads of academic responsibilities when I started my research work. Despite of that, her involvement in each and every protocol being designed, in each and every report that has been documented is stunning. Her excellency, dedication and selflessness as a teacher continue to inspire others particularly the young to become successful mentors and teachers for lifetime. Her vision in promoting research especially among young married women is astonishing. She says, it is never too late to pursue true passions. Her zeal, timelines and never-say-no attitude when approached for even small doubts and questions leaves everyone in awe. I thank her for her patience, faith and understanding in all my endeavors.

A warm thanks to the Principal **Dr. D. Gladis**, MCA., M.Phil., Ph.D., **Mrs. Latha Fenn**, M.Com., M.Phil., (in-charge) and the former Principals **Dr. G. Parameshwari**, **Mrs. Rijivanuneesa** (in-charge), **Dr. S. Nirmaladevi** and **Dr. R. Sarumathy** for their constant support throughout the research period.

I also thank the faculty members of the Biochemistry Department, **Dr. E. Padmini**, M.Sc., M.Phil., Ph.D., **Dr. K. A. Fathima**, M.Sc., M.Phil., Ph.D., **Dr. M. Premalatha**, M.Sc., M.Phil., Ph.D., **Dr. K. Vijayalakshmi**, M.Sc.,Ph.D., **Dr. N. Meenakshi**, M.Sc., Ph.D., and **Mrs. B. Chitra**, M.Sc., and the guest lecturers **Dr. Amutha Ganesh**, M.Sc., M.Phil., Ph.D., **Dr. Sathyadevi**, M.Sc., M.Phil., Ph.D., **Mrs. Varalakshmi**, M.Sc., M.Phil., and **Dr. Kalyani**, M.Sc., M.Phil.,Ph.D., for their help and support during the study.

I would like to thank my doctoral committee members **Dr.K.Vijayalakshmi**, Associate Professor, Department of Biochemistry, Bharathi Women's College, Chennai and **Dr. A. J. Vanisree**, Assistant Professor, University of Madras, Guindy Campus, Chennai for their comments and suggestions for the betterment of research work.

I also thank the non-teaching assistants, **Mr. M. Subramanian, Mr. K. Srinivasan**, **Mr. Loganathan**, **Mr. Vasu**, **Mr. Pazhani**, **Mrs. Lakshmiamma, Mrs. Vasanthi and Mrs. Selvi** who were always there for me for their quick help, and for laboratory care and maintanence.

I express my special thanks to my lovable seniors **Dr. P. Monika, Dr. B. Thendral Hepsibha**, M.Sc., M.Phil., Ph.D., **Dr. Kavitha Yuvaraj**, M.Sc., **Dr. S. Rajapriya**, M.Sc., M.Phil., Ph.D., and **Dr. E.P. Sabina**, M.Sc., M.Phil., Ph.D., and **T.A.K. Mumtaz Begum,** M.Sc., M.Phil., **Ms. R. Rohini Meera**, M.Sc., M.Phil., for their encouragement and timely support during the entire research period.

I express my sincere thanks to **Dr. P. Jayaraman** for plant authentication. I greatly thank the unforgettable efforts by **Dr. K.G Kripa**, Professor, Department of Biochemistry, Vel's University and **Dr. Santhosh Venugopalan**, Head, Department of Pharmacology, Vel's University, during the journey of obtaining ethical clearance for the proposed study.

I would want to acknowledge the support received from **Dr. Palanimuthu** and **Mr. Palanivel** during qPCR analysis, **Mrs. Geetha**, Quality Control Manager, A toZ lab Ambattur, Chennai, during HPLC analysis, **Mr. R. Sathyamoorthi**, Technician, SAIF, IIT-Madras, GC-MS analysis. I thank **Mr. Senthil Kumar,** TANUVAS, Vepery and **Dr. Susruthan Murali**, MBBS., MD., Pathology, Susrutha Diagnostics, Porur, Chennai , during histopathological study.

I would like to express my personal appreciation for the kind and gentle people of my life- my parents, parents-in-law, husband and daughter and all other beloved family members who encouraged me to go on every adventure I take as always. I could not forget their endless love, sacrifices, prayers and support during the research period.

LIST OF ABBREVIATIONS

ABTS	-	2,2'-azino-bis(3-ethylbenzothiazoline-6-sulfonic acid)
DTNB	-	5,5′-dithiobis-(2-nitrobenzoic acid
ATP	-	Adenosine triphosphate
EtOH	-	Alcohol/ Ethanol
BSA	-	Bovine serum albumin
Ca2+	-	Calcium
CEL	-	Carboxyl ester lipase
CPA1	-	Carboxypeptidase A1
CHOP	-	CCAAT-enhancer-binding protein homologous protein
Cer	-	Cerulein
CCK	-	Cholecystokinin
CP	-	Chronic pancreatitis
CTRC	-	Chymotrypsin C
CBB	-	Coomassie brilliant blue
CFTR	-	Cystic fibrosis transmembrane conductance regulator
CFTR	-	Cystic fibrosis transmembrane conductance regulator
CYP2E1	-	Cytochrome P450 2E1
DAMPs	-	Damage associated molecular patterns
DNPH	-	Dinitro phenyl hydrazine
ER	-	Endoplasmic reticulum
FAEE	-	Fatty acid ethyl esters
FOX2	-	Ferrous oxidation xylenol orange
GRP78	-	Glucose-regulated protein
GZ	-	Glycyrrhizin
IκB	-	Inhibitor of nuclear factor kappa B
MDA	-	Malondialdehyde
NIST	-	National Institute of Standards and Technology
NAD^+	-	Nicotinamide adenine dinucleotide

NBT	-	Nitroblue tetrazolium
NF-kB	-	Nuclear factor-kB
OECD	-	Organisation for Economic Co-operation and Development
PAEE	-	Palmitic acid ethyl esters
PMS	-	Phenazonium methosulphate
PBS	-	Phosphate-buffered saline
ROS	-	Reactive oxygen species
SOP	-	Standard operating procedure
TBA	-	Thiobarbituric acid
TIGAR-O	-	Toxic-metabolic, Idiopathic, Genetic, Autoimmune, Recurrent and severe acute pancreatitis, or Obstructive
TCA	-	Trichloroacetic acid
UPR	-	Unfolded protein response
NLRP3	-	NOD-like receptor protein 3/NLR family pyrin domain containing 3
SPINK1	-	Serine protease inhibitor kazal type 1
XBP1	-	X-box binding protein 1
PRSS1&2	-	Serine protease 1&2
ATF4	-	Activating transcription factor 4

LIST OF CHEMICAL FORMULAE

CH3COOH	-	Acetic acid
C2H5OH	-	Alcohol
DH2O	-	Distilled water
HCl	-	Hydrochloric acid
H2O2	-	Hydrogen peroxide
MgCl2	-	Magnesium chloride
C14H16N2	-	Orthotolidine
H3PO4	-	Phosphoric acid
H3PW12O40	-	Phosphotungstic acid
C6H3N3O7	-	Picric acid
K2Cr2O7	-	Potassium dichromate
C3H3NaO3	-	Sodium pyruvate
Na2WO4	-	Sodium tungstate
NaOH	-	Sodiumhydroxide
H2SO4	-	Sulphuric acid
H2SO4	-	Sulphuric acid
CH4N2S	-	Thiourea
C2HCl3O2	-	Trichloroacetic acid

LIST OF FIGURES

LIST OF TABLES

CONTENTS

1. INTRODUCTION

1.1 The gastrointestinal tract

The human digestive system that extends from mouth to anus, includes the gastrointestinal (GI) tract and accessory organs. The GI tract is composed of mouth, pharynx, esophagus, stomach, small and large intestines, rectum and anus. Associated with the GI tract are the following accessory organs: salivary glands, liver, gallbladder, and pancreas. Digestion and absorption of ingested nutrients, and excretion of waste products of digestion are the prime functions of GI tract. Digestion breaks down large macromolecules like proteins, fats and carbohydrates into smaller molecules like amino acids, fatty acids and glucose, that can be absorbed easily and can be used for energy, growth, and cell repair.

1.2 Pancreas

Pancreas is a long and slender glandular organ located behind the stomach, in the retroperitoneal space. The recorded average weight of adult human pancreas is about 100 g and is approximately 14-25cm in length [Atkinson MA,2020]. Pancreas is a heterocrine gland, and it holds both exocrine (pancreatic acinus) and endocrine tissue (pancreatic islet) along with pancreatic ductal cells. Exocrine pancreas is structurally similar to salivary glands and has acinar cells with many zymogen granules, which constitute nearly 85% of the pancreas **(Figure 1.1)**. These zymogen granules contain precursors of the pancreatic enzymes responsible for the digestion of major dietary components. The pancreatic amylase catalyzes the hydrolysis of α-1,4-glucosidic bonds in starch and glycogen. The pancreatic peptidases trypsin, chymotrypsin, and carboxypeptidase A and B and lipases hydrolyse dietary proteins and triglycerides respectively. All these secretions were controlled by neural and hormonal mechanisms. When food reaches the duodenum, enteroendocrine cells release the hormones secretin and cholecystokinin(CCK) into the bloodstream. These hormones stimulate the pancreas to produce large amounts of water, bicarbonate; digestive enzymes amylase and lipase; zymogens trypsinogen, chymotrypsinogen, proelastase and procarboxypeptidase.

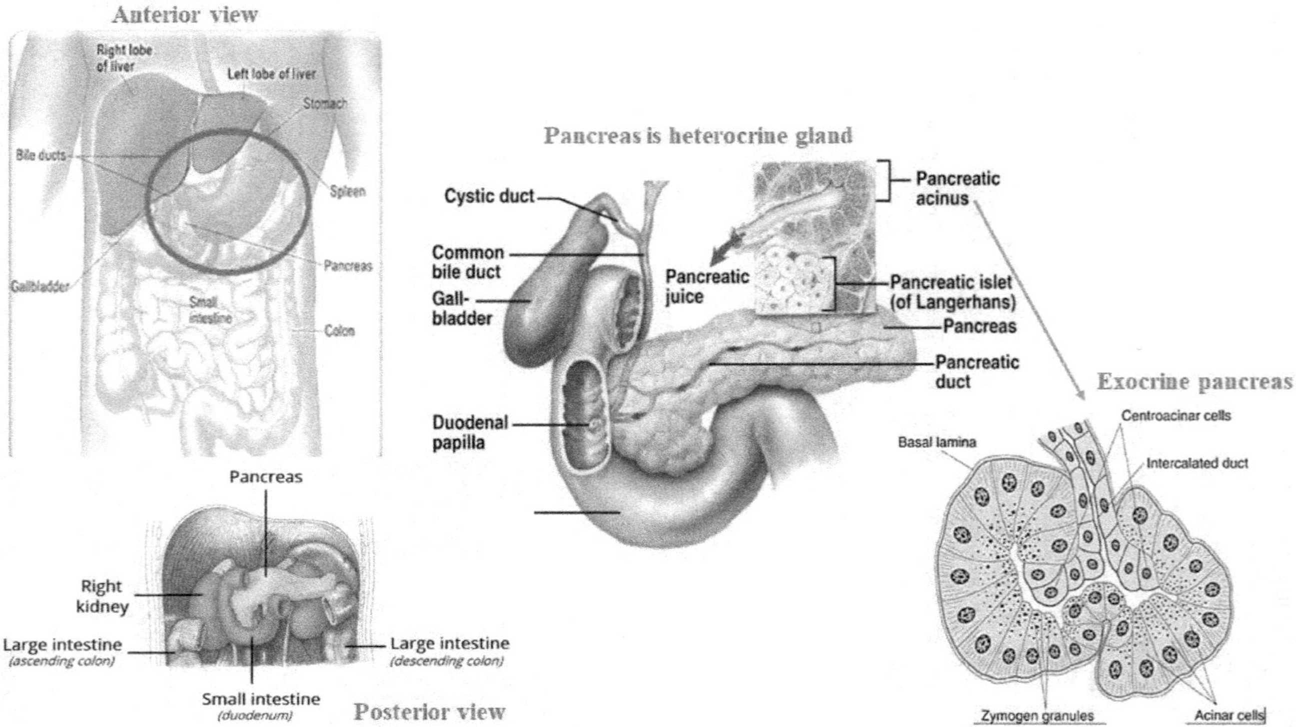

Figure 1.1 Location and anatomy of Pancreas

Inactive enzyme precursors are activated by proteolytic enzymes once they are secreted and are critically important in the digestion of food that enters the small intestine from the stomach. Pancreatic ductal cells secrete huge volumes of bicarbonate-containing fluid and forming a channel for exocrine pancreatic secretions. Endocrine pancreas has islets of Langerhans cells which secrete several hormones like insulin, glucagon, somatostatin and pancreatic polypeptide. It primarily regulates blood glucose levels.

1.3 Common disorders of pancreas

Exocrine pancreatic insufficiency and pancreatitis are major disorders of the pancreas besides diabetes, cystic fibrosis and pancreatic cancer. The common symptoms of malfunctioned pancreas are tenderness, swelling or pain in the abdomen, nausea or vomiting, diarrhea, malnutrition and weight loss.

1.3.1 Exocrine pancreatic insufficiency

Exocrine pancreatic insufficiency (EPI) is a clinical condition, which is characterized by inadequate secretion of pancreatic enzymes by exocrine pancreas, resulting in the inability to digest food properly, or maldigestion [Perbtani Y,2019]. Chronic pancreatitis(CP), pancreatic malignancy, cystic fibrosis, pancreatic resection also has EPI as a consequence.

1.3.2 Diabetes mellitus

Diabetes mellitus (DM) is a disease clinically characterized by chronically elevated blood glucose levels. Diabetes was of three major types-type 1 diabetes mellitus, type 2 diabetes mellitus and gestational diabetes.DM caused as a result of pancreatic diseases is termed as pancraetogenic diabetes or T3cDM or diabetes of exocrine pancreas. T3cDM is as a result of pancreatic inflammation and fibrosis of pancreatic islet cells. But, clinical symptoms are usually observed when more than 90% of exocrine pancreatic functions have declined [Bhattamisra SK,2019].

1.3.3 Cystic fibrosis

Cystic fibrosis, primarily arises due to genetic mutations in the CFTR. It has a wide disease spectrum with recurrent respiratory infections and pancreatic insufficiency as major complications. The small tubes responsible for transporting pancreatic enzymes out of the pancreas are blocked with mucus in cystic fibrosis. The enzymatic build up inside the pancreas instead of digestive system causes pancreatic inflammation [De Boeck K,2020].

1.3.4 Pancreatic cancer

Pancreatic cancer is a highly fatal human cancer type, with a five-year relative survival rate of 8%. Pancreatic cancer is the seventh leading cause of cancer-related deaths worldwide. A long-term inflammation of the pancreas, heavy alcohol consumption, smoking tobacco and nicotine leads to pancreatic cancers along with various inherited gene mutations PRSS1, NF1, BRCA2, p16 [Yao W,2020]. Pancreatic cancer, developing in the exocrine glands of pancreas is termed as pancreatic adenocarcinoma. It is the most common (85%) type which lacks early symptoms. Pancreatic cancer is often diagnosed at an advanced stage [Rawla P,2019].

1.4 Pancreatitis

If the activation of digestive enzymes occurs inside the pancreas itself before they are released into the small intestine, pancreatic digestion and damage is induced and an inflammatory condition called pancreatitis is caused. Different types and causes of pancreatitis were identified like genetic mutations as in hereditary CP, autoimmunity and excessive production of the parathyroid hormone with major risk factors being alcohol, smoking, genetic alterations (pathogenic mutations in genes like CEL, CFTR, CPA1, CTRC, PRSS1, SPINK1) and obesity [Vonlaufen A,2007] [Hegyi P,2020]. Pancreatitis can be acute or chronic. Acute pancreatitis(AP) is necro-inflammatory in nature and is characterized by severe epigastric pain, nausea, vomiting and possibly jaundice [Boxhoorn L,2021]. The most common causes of acute pancreatitis include gallstones and alcohol abuse. Chronic pancreatitis(CP) is a progressive inflammatory condition that causes permanent structural damage in due course. CP results from recurrent episodes of AP, leading to the development of pancreatic insufficiency, steatorrhea, diabetes, pancreatic calcification, and fibrosis. CP can even occur asymptomatically until the emergence of pancreatic insufficiency [Klochkov A,2020]. Numerous evidences have shown that, longterm pre-existing CP as a major risk factor for pancreatic cancer **(Figure 1.2)** [Rawla P,2019].

1.4.1 Causes of chronic pancreatitis:

Etiology behind CP, according to TIGAR-O Classification System is as follows:

Toxic and metabolic causes: Alcohol abuse and smoking act as possible risk factors or important cofactors for CP. Hypercalcemia, hyperparathyroidism, hypertriglyceridemia and organotin compounds like di-n-butyltindichloride (DBTC) are the other known causes for CP. Various medications like antibiotics, psychiatric medications, anti-convulsants, non-steroidal anti-inflammatory medications, chemotherapeutic agents, anti-lipemics, anti-hypertensives, anti-hyperglycemics, and various anti-viral agents were reported to cause drug-induced pancreatitis [Nitsche C,2012].

Idiopathic causes: There exist two forms of idiopathic CP- Early onset, Late onset and Tropical CP. The exact reason behind this CP is not known [Midha S,2010].

***Genetic causes**:* Anionic trypsinogen PRSS2, Autosomal recessive /modifier genes, CFTR mutations, SPINK1 mutations, cationic trypsinogen (codon 16, 22, 23 mutations), a1-antitrypsin deficiency (possible), monocyte chemoprotectant protein [LaRusch J,2011].

Autoimmune etiology: Isolated/associated with other autoimmune disorders.

Recurrent and severe acute pancreatitis: There exists a strong association between recurrent acute and chronic pancreatitis as reported from different clinicopathological and animal studies [Etemad B,2001].

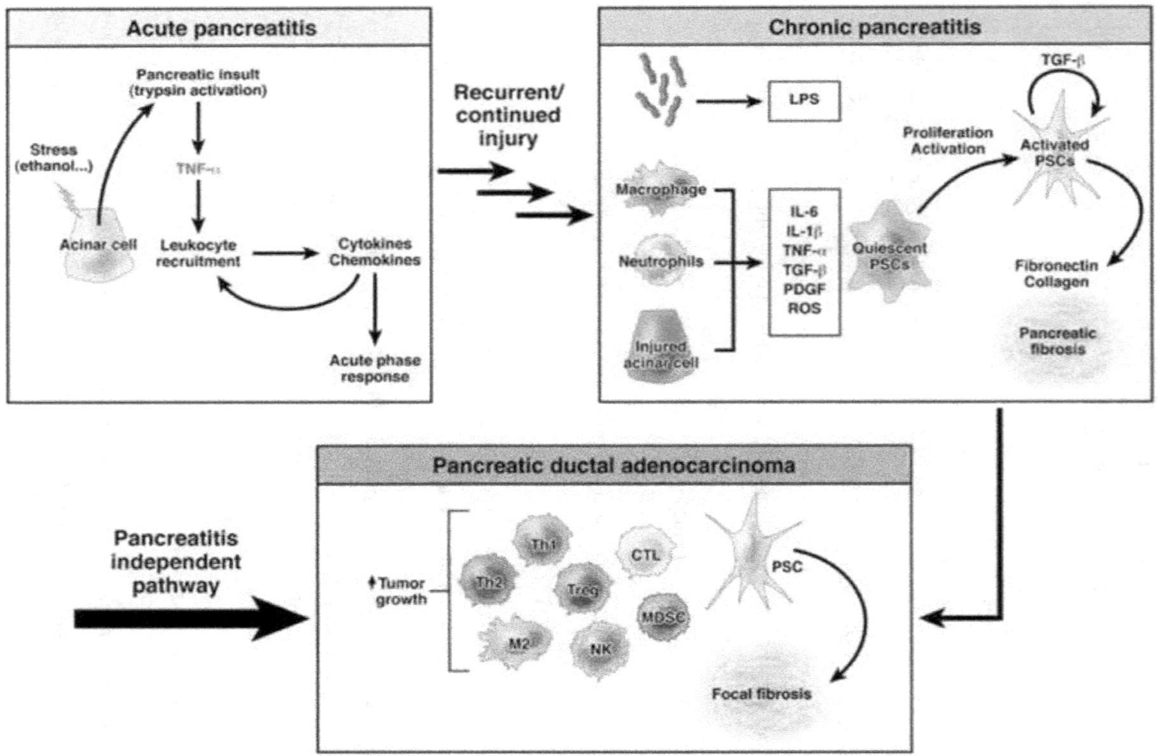

Figure 1.2 Prior history of pancreatitis accelerates pancreatic adenocarcinoma
(Source: https://www.gastrojournal.org/article/S0016-5085(13)00197-2/)

Obstructive etiology: Gallstones, Pancreatic divisum, Sphincter of Oddi disorders, Duct obstruction by tumors and lesions, Choledochal cysts and abnormal pancreatobiliary unions and Inflammatory bowel disease **(Figure 1.3)** [Majumder S,2016].

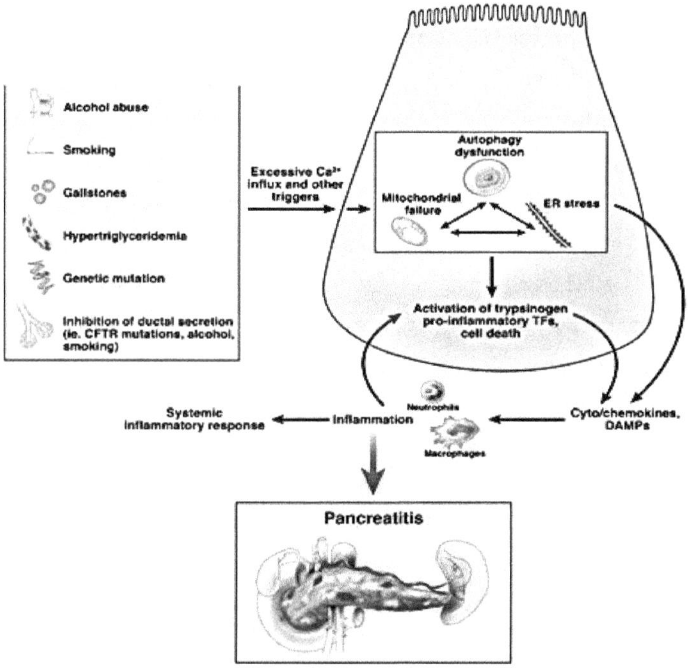

Figure 1.3 Causes and pathological consequences of CP
(Source: https://pubmed.ncbi.nlm.nih.gov/30660726/)

1.4.2 Symptoms of chronic pancreatitis

The major cardinal symptoms of CP are Abdominal pain, Steatorrhea and Weight loss.

Abdominal Pain: Severe and disabling abdominal pain is the hallmark of CP and is the most commonly (40%) reported reason, behind hospitalization in CP patients. Structural abnormalities causing ductal hypertension, might be the underlying morphological changes for causing clinical pain [Wehler M,2004]. It can be continuous pain or relapsing pain. As food intake can trigger pain exacerbations, patients usually respond by reducing food consumption. This can lead to progressive weight loss and malnutrition. In some patients (5.8% to 20%), CP can be basically painless, with exocrine and endocrine insufficiency alone as major symptom.

Exocrine and endocrine insufficiency: Severe exocrine insufficiency is the common symptom (86.6%) at the time of diagnosis, compared to endocrine insufficiency in CP. Exocrine insufficiency results from reduced digestive enzyme output and decreased bicarbonate secretion, caused because of progressive destruction of pancreatic tissue. Typical symptoms of exocrine insufficiency are cramps, gas, bloating, flatulence and steatorrhea. Nutrient malabsorption and weight loss caused due to pancreatic exocrine insufficiency, always exists in CP. Endocrine insufficiency leads to complications like diabetes mellitus secondary to CP. Rarely this pancreatogenic diabetes leads to diabetic retinopathy. Nondiabetic retinal lesions and retinal function abnormalities were also reported in CP patients [Toskes PP,1979]. The organ reserve of pancreas is so large that the symptoms become evident only in the advanced conditions of CP [Keller J,2015].

Steatorrhea: Steatorrhea is the very early symptom observed in CP and is more severe than malabsorption. Steatorrhea is clinically excretion of voluminous, fatty stools because of excessive discharge of nitrogenous substances in the feces, when pancreatic lipase secretions are disturbed [Vincent D,2004].

1.4.3 Experimental pancreatitis

1.4.3.1 Alcoholic pancreatitis

Prolonged alcohol (EtOH) administration fails to produce CP in animal models, despite alcohol being a major risk factor of CP [Gukovsky I,2008]. In previous experimental animal studies, chronic alcohol exposure at very high doses or as liquid diet or as continuous intragastric infusions did not result in a pronounced injury to the pancreas [Deng X,2005]. Rather than CP, only mild functional insufficiencies were documented. But, alcohol sensitizes pancreas to injury by other triggers, which cause initiation of this disease. Due to its high influence on pancreatic pathology, alcohol was still chosen as one of the triggers for CP in animal models. Alcohol feeding to rats, when combined with triggers like caerulein injections, the course of pancreatitis is exacerbated with increase in calcifications, pancreatic fibrosis and loss of parenchyma in animal models [Aghdassi AA,2011].

1.4.3.2 Cerulein pancreatitis

The peptide hormone CCK and its analog cerulein(Cer) were used with in vitro models to reproducibly induce acute pancreatitis-like disease response in pancreatic acinar cells. The most widely adopted animal model of CP is repetitive cerulein injection [Reed A,2014]. Physiologically, CCK plays a pivotal role in regulating exocrine secretions of pancreas, after stimulation by food ingestion. Cerulein is an analog of cholecystokinin-8 (CCK-8) **(Figure 1.4)** that acts on CCK receptors and elicit recurring episodes of acute pancreatitis by hyper stimulation of exocrine pancreas in rats. Rats when chronically fed alcohol, have an increased sensitivity to recurring episodes of acute pancreatitis induced by cerulein facilitating the progression to chronic pathological changes as in human alcoholic CP [Lampel M,1977].

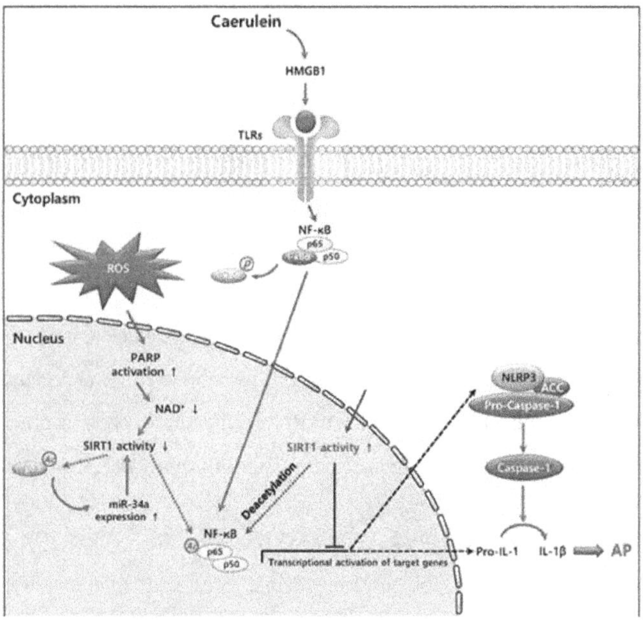

Figure 1.4 Role of cerulein in eliciting pancreatitis

(Source: https://www.nature.com/articles/s41598-017-03418-0)

It has been proved that, such an acute pancreatitis event also causes recruitment of inflammatory cells, fibrosis and oxidative stress in pancreas resulting in chronic pathological changes in pancreas. And the EtOH and Cer induced pancreatitis model is proved to recapitulate similar pathology of CP in human beings including fibrosis and chronic inflammation [Deng X,2005]. It is a well-accepted, non-invasive, time-dependent and highly reproducible model.

1.4.4 Pathophysiology of chronic pancreatitis

1.4.4.1 Effect of alcohol in CP

Alcohol abuse is the primary and definitive cause of CP, resulting in approximately 40 to 70% of all cases. It increases the risk of developing pancreatic cancer by 20 times.

Direct toxic effects: Alcohol is known to show its deleterious effect on spincter of oddi, cause precipitation by increasing the viscosity of pancreatic secretions, leading to the formation of protein plugs and calculi inside the small ducts. This causes ulceration, scarring, subsequent acinar cell atrophy and fibrosis [Vonlaufen A,2007].

Effect on acinar cells: Alcohol causes increased synthesis of digestive and lysosomal enzymes. It is accompanied by decreased exocytosis and increased membrane fragility of lysosomal and zymogen granules, thus predisposing the acinar cell to activate intracellular enzymes prematurely and auto digest. Alcohol also cause acinar cell damage as subcellular membranes, proteins, and nucleic acids were attacked by reactive oxygen species(ROS) of ethanol metabolism. Alcohol causes elevations in intracellular calcium (Ca2+) leading to mitochondrial depolarization and cell death. Release of cytokines by injured acinar cells, can damage adjacent cells.

Effect on pancreatic stellate cells (PSCs): Activation of PSCs by ethanol and its metabolites and by cytokines from acinar cells and inflammatory cells, leads to progressive fibrosis [Apte MV,2010] **(Figure 1.5)**.

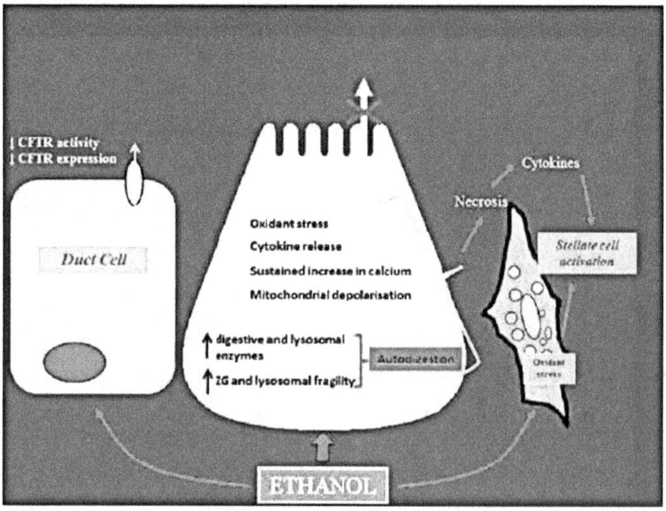

Figure 1.5 Effect of alcohol on different cells of pancreas

Pancreas is equipped with oxidative and non-oxidative metabolic pathways to process the ingested alcohol. In the oxidative pathway, acetaldehyde formed causes toxic effects on acinar cells through activating of stellate cells, increasing levels of proinflammatory cytokines, and decreasing NAD+/NADH ratio. The oxidative pathway is catalyzed primarily by alcohol dehydrogenase (ADH), minorly by cytochrome P450 2E1 (CYP2E1) and catalase **(Figure 1.6)**.

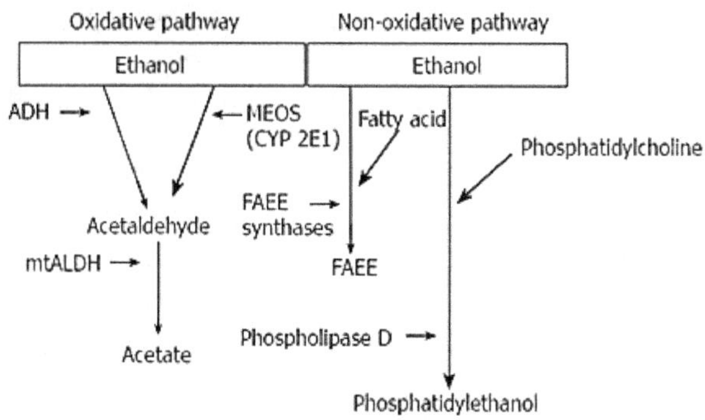

ADH: Alcohol dehydrogenase; mt ALDH: Mitochondrial aldehyde dehydrogenase; FAEE synthase: Fatty acid ethyl ester synthase

Figure 1.6 Metabolism of ethanol

(Source: https://www.wjgnet.com/1007-9327/full/v12/i43/wjg-12-6926-g001.htm)

Generation of excessive ROS takes place during oxidation of ethanol by CYP2E1[Norton ID,1998]. The non-oxidative pathway involves the formation of fatty acid ethyl esters (FAEE). It triggers the activation of key transcription factors, sustained increase in intracellular calcium, ultimately leading to further cell injury. Metabolites of alcohol also initiate recruitment of inflammatory cells and cause fibrosis [Gukovsky I,2008]. Besides, alcohol is responsible for premature activation of trypsinogen and other digestive enzymes within the acinar cells itself; causing the pancreatic tissue to auto-digest and even accelerating inflammation. Activation of nuclear factor-kB (NF-kB), which is a central transcription regulator of inflammation, by alcohol and ROS further propels the entire inflammatory response causing about 50% of pancreatic tissue damage [Gukovskaya AS,2004] **(Figure 1.7)**.

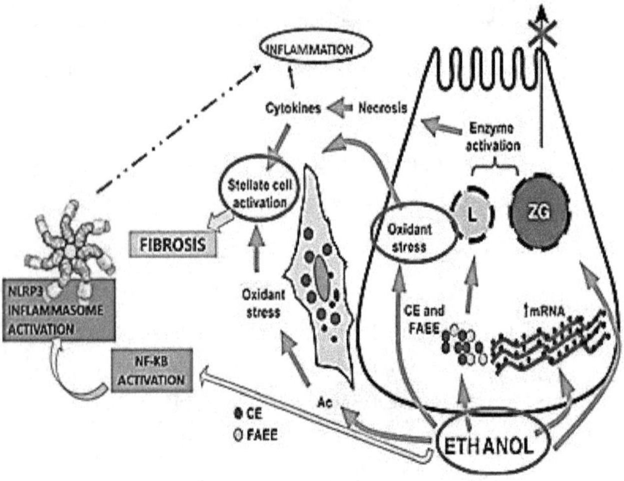

Figure 1.7 Toxic effects of alcohol on the pancreatic acinar cells

1.4.4.2 Oxidative stress in alcohol and cerulein induced pancreatitis:

Oxidative stress is very important pathological event in CP. Xenobiotics like alcohol and nicotine are detoxified in the body through phase I and phase II pathways chiefly in the liver and partly in pancreas. Overwhelmed alcohol detoxification by CYP2E1, which is a phase-1 metabolic clearance enzyme, results in increased ROS and oxidative stress condition in pancreas [Telek G,2001] [Apte MV, 1998]. Chronic oxidative stress leads to fibrosis. Oxidative stress extends both clinical and histological symptoms of CP like pain and fibrosis-necrosis events respectively, causing disease progression [Bhardwaj P,2013].

Increased NADH supply to pancreatic mitochondria during intensified alcohol metabolism, activated xanthine oxidase produced by damaged pancreas, NADPH oxidase of PSCs, recruited inflammatory PMN leucocytes, cytochrome P450 were the estimated sources of pathogenic oxidative stress, basically creating overwhelmed ROS production during pancreatitis [Shalbueva N,2013] [Folch E,1998] [Masamune A,2008].

In response to pancreatic injury, an inflammatory process is also initiated in pancreas, that leads to the recruitment of innate immune cells like neutrophils and macrophages towards the site of pancreatic injury. First, recruitment of neutrophils and monocytes takes place, followed by dendritic cells, mast cells, T cells, and platelets [Sandoval DI,1996]. Immune cells play a major role in the pancreatic pathology. Neutrophils are not usually present in healthy pancreas. Neutrophils are also the prime sources of ROS production [Gukovskaya AS,2017]. The immune cell infiltration in association with injured pancreatic acinar cells, produce more cytokines and chemokines exaggerating the inflammatory response inside the pancreas. ROS, along with proteases and growth factors released by neutrophils and macrophages cause tissue damage, besides fibroblast proliferation. ROS also serves as a potent molecular trigger of various inflammatory mechanisms. ROS can instantly attack biological membranes, stimulating arachidonic acid metabolism with increased production of prostaglandins, thromboxanes, and leukotrienes. Furthermore, with its chemoattractant nature ROS triggers neutrophil aggregation and their subsequent adherence to the capillary walls [Kim H,2008].

Hence it is possible that, ROS play a central role in the prolonging pancreatic inflammation and development of extrapancreatic complications [Tsai K,1998]. In brief, CP results in oxidative stress which amplifies the inflammatory process.

1.4.4.3 Role of Inflammation in CP

Tissue injury caused to pancreatic acinar cells by various pancreatic insults, leads to the release of damage associated molecular patterns (DAMPs), which are the endogenous molecules of the host: nuclear proteins like histones and high mobility group box-1 (HMGB1), nuclear and mitochondrial DNA, heat shock proteins (HSP) and adenosine triphosphate (ATP). DAMPs can initiate sterile inflammation in pancreas [Kang R,2014]. The other probable means by which damaged acinar cells induce inflammation is, by triggering the synthesis and release of cytokines, chemokines and intercellular adhesion molecule-1(ICAM-1). Consequently, infiltration of neutrophils and monocytes takes place at the site of tissue injury.

The major pathway responsible for the pancreatitis disease severity and progression is NF-κB activation. NF-kB is the pleiotropic transcription factor and a key regulator of cytokine induction. Unlike other transcription factors, NF-κB is retained inactive in the cytoplasm, along with its inhibitors named as IκB proteins. The process of sequestration prevents nuclear migration of NF-κB, its DNA binding and further activation. In response to stimuli, the IκBs are phosphorylated by IκB kinases on serine residues in specific, resulting in IκB ubiquitylation and proteasome-mediated degradation. This allows nuclear translocation of NF-κB, initiating cytokine expression **(Figure 1.8)**. Excess ROS, in response to ethanol and cerulein could activate IκB kinase and NF-κB [Kim H,2008]. Cerulein hyperstimulation was shown to cause degradation of IκB, causing direct NF-κB activation in pancreatic acinar cells. Blocking of NF-kB activation improves rat cerulein pancreatitis [Gukovsky I,1998].

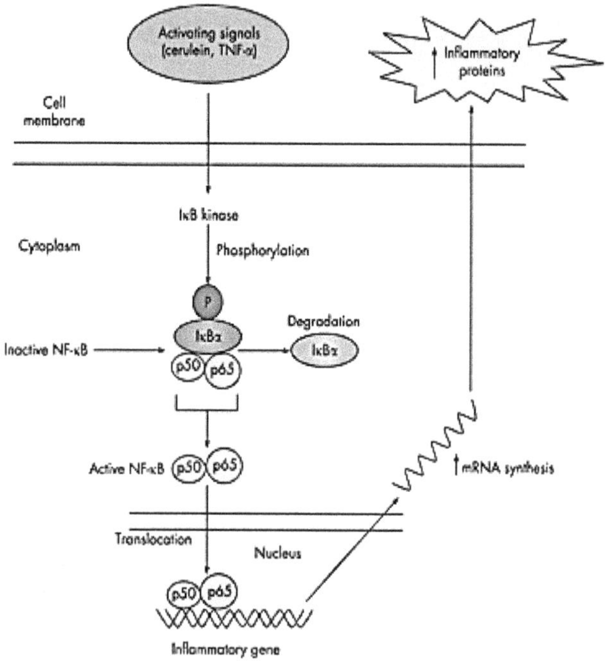

Figure 1.8 Activation of NF-κB
(Source: https://gut.bmj.com/content/57/2/259)

Ethanol metabolism by CYP2E1 produces excess ROS which activates NF-κB, that is very sensitive to ROS [Kim H,2008]. ROS prompts pro-inflamamtory cytokine signalling through NF-κB pathway. DAMPs, ROS, acetaldehyde and FAEEs were reported to activate NF-κB in CP. Ethanol also induces inflammatory response through NF-κB activation [Gukovskaya AS,2004]. Cerulein causes NF-κB activation by enhancing ROS production through NADPH oxidase [Kim H,2008].

Rheumatoid arthritis, atherosclerosis, COPD, asthma, multiple sclerosis, inflammatory bowel disease and ulcerative colitis are the other chronic inflammatory diseases associated with NF-κB activation [Lawrence T,2009].

1.4.4.4 Inflammasomes

Inflammasomes are multiprotein complexes belonging to innate immune system, consisting of a sensor protein, inflammatory caspases, and sometimes an adjoining adapter protein. They can be activated by a variety of endogenous and exogenous stimuli, leading to enzymatic activation of canonical caspase-1, noncanonical caspase-11. This results in the secretion of IL-1β and IL-18, as well as apoptotic and pyroptotic cell death pathways. Proper inflammasome activation is very essential for the host to combat invading pathogens or tissue damages, while devastating inflammasome activation leads to unrestricted tissue responses contributing to diversified inflammatory, metabolic and neurodegenerative disorders [Zheng D,2020].

Factors that elicit an innate inflammatory response inside host cells can be classified as pathogen-associated molecular patterns (PAMPs): which are conserved components of infectious agents, and damage-associated molecular patterns (DAMPs): which are stress signals from the host itself. PAMPs and DAMPs are sensed by variety of pattern recognition receptors (PRRs) and cells of innate and adaptive immunity [Schroder K,2010].

Many cytoplasmic PRRs are capable of assembling into an inflammasome complex and are named according to their protein domains. NBD leucine-rich repeat-containing receptor (NLR) family contains subfamilies distinguished by their N-terminal effector domains. There exists four recognizable NLR N-terminal domains: the acidic transactivation domain, pyrin domain, caspase recruitment domain (CARD), and baculoviral inhibitory repeat (BIR)-like domains. Inflammasome-assembling PRRs are present mainly in macrophages, neutrophils and various other immune cells [Martinon F,2009].

Inflammasome signaling culminates in inflammatory caspase-activation. Assembly of a hetero-oligomeric complex: NOD-like receptor-pyrin-containing proteins (NLRP) or AIM2 protein, and sometimes the additional adapter and effector protein: apoptosis-associated speck-like protein containing a CARD (ASC) is required **(Figure 1.9)**. The activation of caspases results in the proteolytic activation of the proinflammatory cytokines interleukin-1β and/or interleukin-18, both of which are immensely involved in activation and regulation of inflammation [Strowig T,2012].

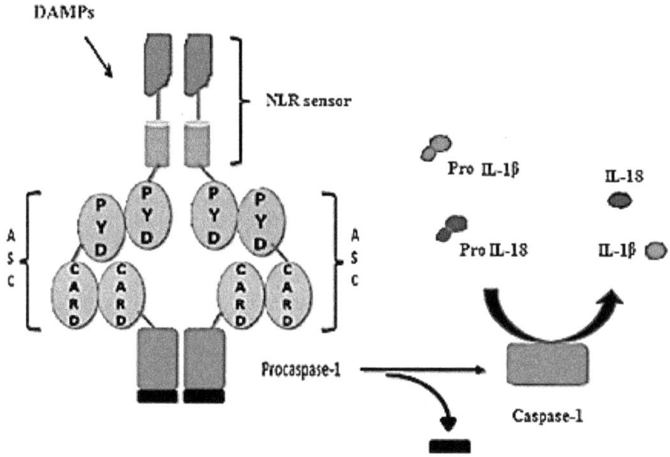

DAMPs: Damage associated molecular patterns, **NLR:** Nod-like receptor, **PYD:** Pyrin domain, **CARD:** Caspase recruitment domain, **ASC:** Adapter apoptosis-associated speck-like protein, **IL:** Interleukin

Figure 1.9 Components of inflammasome

1.4.4.5 ER in alcoholic CP

The prime role of exocrine pancreas is to produce digestive enzymes. The pancreatic acinar cell synthesizes, stores, and secretes the proenzymes and enzymes needed to digest dietary proteins, carbohydrates, and lipids. To facilitate these functions, pancreatic acinar cell has very high rates of protein synthesis and abundant endoplasmic reticulum(ER). ER requires balanced redox conditions and calcium concentrations to achieve such a functional status. Furthermore, ER itself is a major intracellular calcium store. Nascent proteins will be folded, modified, and sent to secretory (zymogen) granules. Physiologically, meal intake stimulates neural and hormonal pathways, which cause exocytosis by zymogen granules of acinar cell into the pancreatic duct [Cooley MM,2020].

Ordered protein folding and their transport to the secretory pathway was completely disrupted under the influence of alcohol and alcohol induced-oxidative stress, stimulating an adaptive pathway called ER stress in pancreas **(Figure 1.10)**. Numerous reports have brought to light that, disruption in ER functions is associated with AP and CP [Waldron RT,2018]. Disturbances in protein folding induces a stress response called unfolded protein response (UPR), to mitigate ER stress.

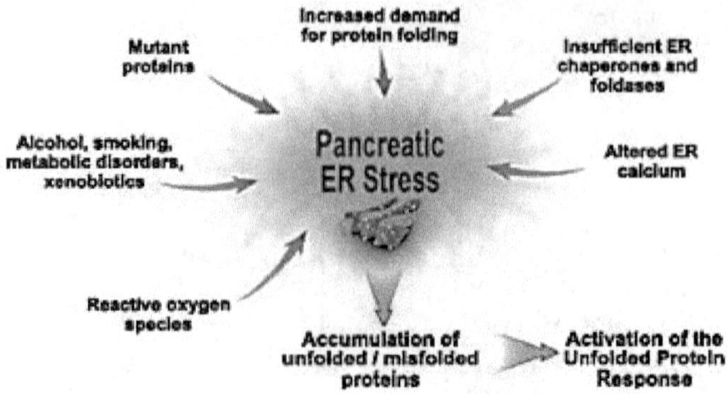

Figure 1.10 **ER stress in pancreas**

(Source: https://www.frontiersin.org/articles/10.3389/fphys.2011.00008/full)

It involves various UPR transcription factors like protein kinase RNA-like endoplasmic reticulum kinase (PERK), activating transcription factor 6 (ATF6) and inositol-requiring enzyme 1 (IRE1), which are transmembrane proteins. In general, these proteins are kept inactive by a 78 kDa, glucose-regulated protein (GRP78). GRP78/BiP is a master regulator chaperone of UPR. Their downstream signaling factors include activating transcription factor 4 (ATF4), CCAAT-enhancer-binding protein homologous protein (CHOP) and X-box binding protein 1 (XBP1) which are aimed to restore ER homeostasis **(Figure 1.11)**.

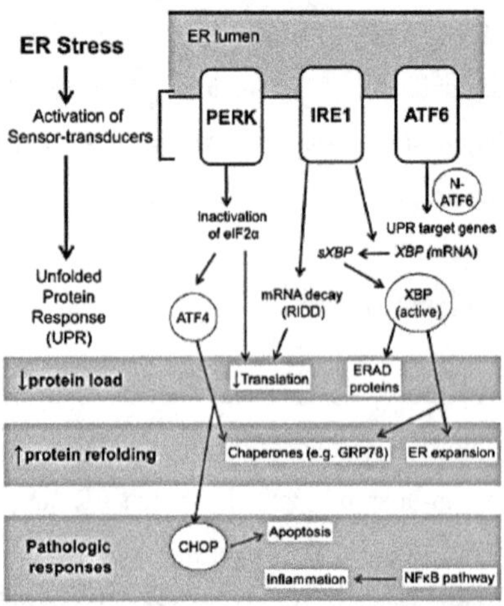

Figure 1.11 **Role of UPR components in ER stress**
(Source: Sah RP, 2014)

The ER stress response in mammals is biphasic: adaptation and apoptosis. Cells firstly adapt to the accumulation of unfolded proteins by inducing ER-resident stress chaperons like GRP78. These proteins initiate refolding of unfolded proteins. But, if there occurs no fruitful adaptation, the apoptotic response is initiated, by both ATF6- and ATF4-dependent activation of CHOP protein [Zinszner H,1998].

ATF6 is transported to the Golgi and then to nucleus, where it induces the expression of various transcription factors regulating, overexpression of UPR components such as ER-associated protein degradation (ERAD) to decrease accumulation of unfolded proteins and ER chaperones with an aim of stabilizing protein folding [Sah RP,2014].Active form of PERK phosphorylates the α subunit of eukaryotic initiation factor 2 (eIF2α) that is in connection with protein translation of ATF4, inducing expression of protein folding factors involved in ER homeostasis. IRE1 is the most conserved modulator of the ER stress signaling pathway and exists in two isoforms, IRE1α and IRE1β.Both of these forms show differences in their tissue expression. IRE1α is expressed in all cell types and under stress conditions; in an active form it catalyzes the splicing of XBP-1 into mature XBP1, involved in the regulation of protein folding [Walter P,2011]. CHOP is the prime chaperone for ER stress-mediated apoptosis. PERK activation induces eIF2 phosphorylation, which inturn activates ATF4, consequently determining the upregulation of proapoptotic factor CHOP. ATF6 also regulates expression of CHOP. Transcriptional targets of CHOP were found to increase cellular ROS and $Ca2+$ levels [Martucciello S,2020]. CHOP promotes expression of inhibitors of apoptosis antagonists such as bcl-2 inturn promoting apoptosis [Walter P,2011].

Unresolved UPR and ER stress leads to failed homeostasis and cytotoxic cellular damage [Lugea A,2015]. Additionally, activation of the highly studied transcription factor of inflammation NF-kB, has been proved to be a consequence of ER stress [Tam AB,2012], and it requires ROS and $Ca2+$ as second messengers [Pahl HL,1996].

1.4.4.6 Mitochondria in alcoholic CP

Mitochondria holds a significant portion of pancreatic acinar cell volume (around 8-10 %) and are the primary sources of ATP production, as acinar cells are the sites for prominent protein synthesis. Various other organelles interact with the ER, and mitochondria are of functionally important among them. ER stress progresses, with the release of calcium into the mitochondria (Marchi S, 2014).

Physiologically, both cytosolic Ca2+ and ER Ca2+ are tightly regulated. Influx of Ca2+ into ER is managed by sarcoplasmic/ER Ca2+ ATPase (SERCA) pumps. In cellular stress, where Ca2+- acts as a signal, Ca2+ is released from ER stores through ryanodine receptors (RyR) and precisely by the IP3Rs. IP3Rs are found present in the MAM regions, where ER and mitochondria are associated Mitochondrial Ca2+ influx is under the control of voltage-dependent anion channel (VDAC), residing on the outer mitochondrial membrane, facilitating Ca2+ transfer between these two organelles [Rizzuto R,1998].

Mitochondrially derived oxidative stress is the key event in various diseases like Parkinson's disease, Alzheimer's disease, besides playing pathological role in aging process and diabetes [Feissner RF,2009]. Pancreatic physiological bioenergetics is disrupted during alcohol and cerulein-induced pancreatitis. Various pathophysiological triggers like fatty acids, reactive oxygen species, and non-oxidative alcohol metabolites can deplete cellular ATP [Shalbueva N,2013]. Physiological concentrations of CCK induce oscillatory Ca2+ responses in acinar cells whereas supraphysiological levels prompt pancreatic acinar cells, to generate local and global Ca2+ transients. Ca2+-induced mitochondrial dysfunction, compromised ATP production and its subsequent necrosis are the important pathological features for the progression of pancreatitis [Javed MA,2018]. It has been previously documented that, PAEE and palmitoleic acid, produced by the hydrolysis of FAEEs induce mitochondrial dysfunction through sustained elevations of cytosolic Ca2+ [Criddle DN,2006]. Opening of mitochondrial permeability transition pore (MPTP) mediates mitochondrial dysfunction in pancreas. The triggers for MPTP opening being sustained elevation of mitochondrial Ca2+ and excessive ROS production [Biczo G,2018]. Restraining excessive ROS with antioxidants and reduction of Ca2+ overload that causes mitochondrial dysfunction could be a potential therapeutic approach in the pancreas. Disturbed bioenergetics is the underlying cause of mitochondrial dysfunction in pancreatitis [Booth DM,2011.

The electron transport chain(ETC) complexes I and III are the prime mitochondrial sources of univalent reduction of O2 into superoxide (O2·−) **(Figure 1.12)**. O2·− is very unstable and fastly reacts with neighbouring molecules, dismutes as hydrogen peroxide (H2O2) and O2, sometimes enzymatically dismuted by the superoxide dismutase (SOD) enzyme family. Unlike O2·−, H2O2 has good membrane permeability. It can in turn react with metal ions forming highly reactive hydroxyl radical (OH·) [Kussmaul L,2006]. Complex-1 is the first major component in the mitochondrial electron transport chain (ETC). It transfers electrons from reduced nicotinamide adenine dinucleotide (NADH) to coenzyme Q leading to ATP synthesis. Complex-1 is the site for the production of ROS and inturn a target of ROS [Clemens, 2014].

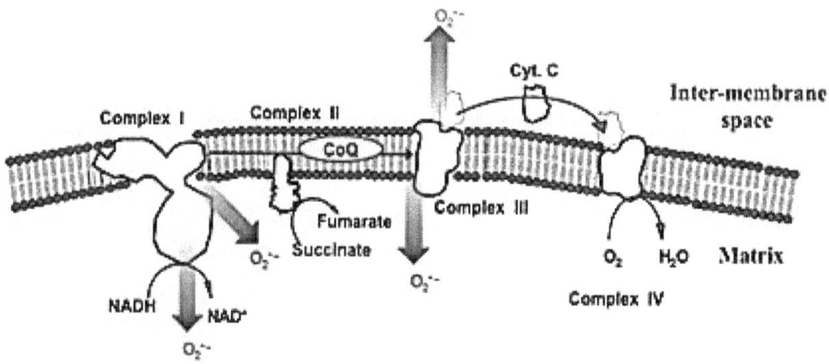

Figure 1.12 Production of ROS (superoxides) during mitochondrial ETC

During ETC, protons flow through ATP synthase, which is located in the inner membrane of mitochondria to drive ATP synthesis. Specifically, electrons are transferred from NADH to oxygen through a series of complexes like NADH-Q reductase (complex I), succinate -Q reductase (complex II), Q-cytochrome c reductase (complex III) and cytochrome c oxidase (complex IV). Mitochondria use large amounts of O2 for the production of energy. As one molecule of O2 is passed through ETC, free radicals like superoxide anions (O2·-), termed as ROS are generated. When excessive ROS are produced, mitochondrial antioxidants cannot scavenge oxidants at an ample rate leading to damaged mitochondrial components and there by mitochondrial oxidative stress. Preventing mitochondrial damage improves several pathological aspects of pancreatitis, ameliorating disease severity [Shalbueva N, 2013].

During alcohol and cerulein-induced pancreatitis, an ROS-generating mitochondrion can activate NLRP3 inflammasome. NLRP3 can confess DAMPs released from damaged mitochondria and serves as signaling platform for the activation of caspase-1 and release of pro-inflammatory cytokines, interleukin-1β and interleukin-18. Mitochondria-induced NLRP3 inflammasome activation is implicated in various inflammatory diseases [Zhou, 2011] [Gurung P, 2015].

1.4.5 Treatment of alcoholic CP

In most cases, patients with CP suffer from intractable and debilitating abdominal pain, that is resistant to analgesic drug regimen. Pancreatic insufficiency and malnutrition are the other prominent symptoms of CP. Currently, there is no specific drug available for CP to reverse its course and progression.

Pancreatic exocrine insufficiency emerges clinically as steatorrhea, weight loss, malnutrition, metabolic bone disease, vitamin and mineral deficiencies. Supportive therapy to combat exocrine and endocrine insufficiencies with pancreatic enzyme supplements and antioxidants besides management of complications like pain is suggested. Antioxidants widely used include selenium, ascorbic acid, β-carotene, and methionine [Kirk GR,2006]. Malnutrition is another primary problem with chronic pancreatitis especially because of the fat maldigestion and malabsorption. Pancreatic enzyme replacement therapy was found effective against fat and protein maldigestion [Min M,2018].

Chronic and persistent abdominal pain associated with CP can reduce quality of life to a great extent. It becomes essential to treat CP soon it is diagnosed, because repeated episodes of inflammation can damage pancreas and pain relief becomes much more less effective. Pain is mostly managed by a combination of analgesics, adjuvant analgesics and opiods with increasing analgesic potency. Opiods have intrinsic effects on gastrointestinal motility besides causing addiction, abuse and tolerance. Non-steroidal anti-inflammatory drugs (NSAIDs) have been shown to act as anti-inflammatory and analgesic agents. NSAIDs are particularly useful but less favorable for their side effects and toxicity to the GI tract including ulcers and bleeding [Sostres C,2010]. An alternative to NSAID therapy is always a better consideration. Lifestyle modifications like complete cessation of alcohol and consuming small, frequent, low-fat meals is suggested. Although narcotics relieve pain, one-half of the patients eventually might require surgery. Use of transdermal fentanyl and sustained-release morphine tablets was also recorded previously in CP. Injection of pharmaceuticals like, a combination of a local anesthetic and a steroid, i.e., bupivacaine and triamcinolone into the celiac ganglia is a common surgical, opiod-free approach for the treatment of CP [Gardner TB,2020].

1.5 Traditional herbal medicines

India is a land of great diversity, a home for a large variety of flora and fauna, and is a land for the emergence of traditional medical folklore like Ayurveda, Homeopathy and Siddha. Various varieties of plant-based traditional systems are in practice in our country. According to WHO, nearly 80% of the world populations still rely on medicinal herbs for their primary health care [Thakkar S,2020]. But making traditional medicine truly mainstream, by incorporating its knowledge into modern healthcare, and ensuring its safety and efficacy standards is not an easy task.

CP can be treated with herbal medicine and with a recommended dietary regimen, which eventually improves digestion bringing down the need for digestive enzyme supplements. Pain is reduced gradually with less chances of recurrence. Emblica officinalis (Indian amla), Nigella sativa (Black cumin), Terminalia chebula (Gall nut), Morus alba (White mulberry), Brasssica olaraeceae (Broccoli) are the scientifically proved wonder herbs for the treatment of CP **(Figure 1.13)**.

And here is an attempt to give one of the nature's treasures a new look. The present study is focused on one such very effective and potent ayurvedic medicinal herb- *Glycyrrhiza glabra* **(Figure 1.14)**.

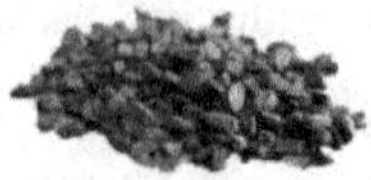

Nigella sativa **(Black cumin)**

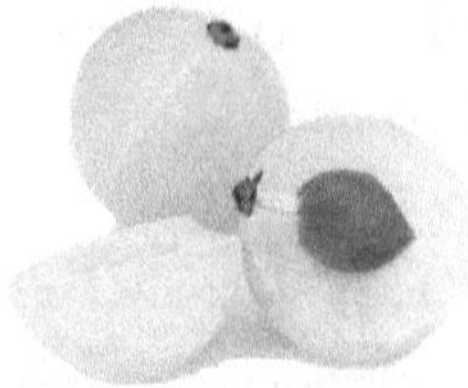

Emblica officinalis **(Gooseberry)**

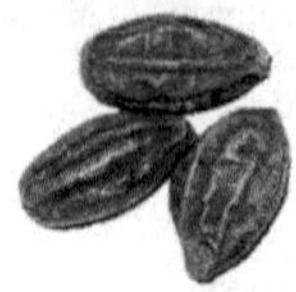

Terminalia chebula **(Myrobalan)**

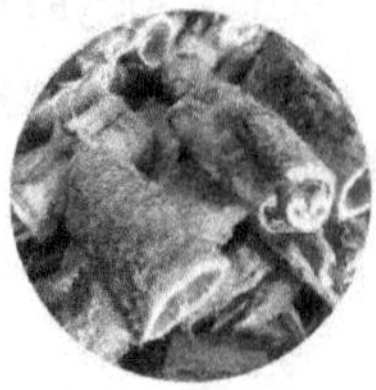

Morus alba **(White mulberry)**

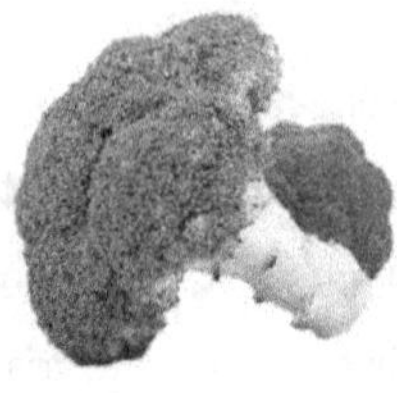

Brassica oleracea **(Broccoli)**

Figure 1.13 Pancreato protective natural sources

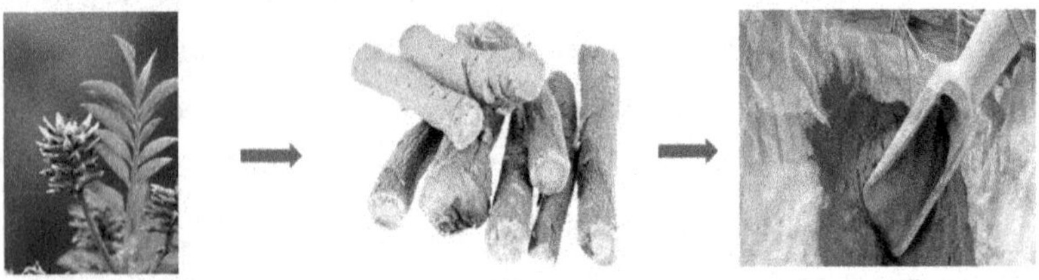

Glycyrrhiza glabra **plant** *Glycyrrhiza glabra* **root** *Glycyrrhiza glabra* **root extract (dried)**

Figure 1.14 ***Glycyrrhiza glabra*** **(Licorice)**

1.5.1 *Glycyrrhiza Glabra*

Glycyrrhiza glabra Linn is one of the most extensively used medicinal herb from the ancient medical history of Ayurveda. The first written documents can be ascertained back to ancient Assyrian, Mediterranean, Egyptian, Chinese, and Indian cultures. The word *Glycyrrhiza* is derived from the Greek term *glykos* (meaning sweet) and *rhiza* (meaning root). *Glycyrrhiza glabra* Linn, commonly known as 'liquorice' and 'sweet wood' belongs to Leguminosae family. It is estimated to be 50-60 times sugarier than sugarcane [Omar HR,2012]. Vernacular names for liquorice are Jeshthamadh (Marathi), Jothi- madh(Hindi),Yashtimadhu,

Madhuka (Sanskrit), Jashtimadhu, Jaishbomodhu (Bengali), Atimadhuram, Yashtimadhukam (Telugu), Jethimadhu (Gujarati) and Atimadhuram (Tamil) [Damle M,2014]. It is commonly used as a flavoring and sweetening herb in candy and baking industries, its tea for thirst quenching, its dried root for cleansing teeth. In beer and fire extinguisher producing industries, the root extracts are used as foaming agents. It is highly recommended for skin depigmentation in cosmetic preparations [Pastorino G,2018]. World Health Organization & Food and Agriculture Organization of the United Nations, during their 63th report on evaluation of food additives, commented the safety aspects of licorice extracts and its natural constituent, glycyrrhizin [Joint FA,2005].

Licorice root decoction, when applied to HaCaT human keratinocyte cell line, it has been shown to augment tumour necrosis factor-α (TNF-α) and interferon-γ-mediated chemokine production by targeting the STAT1 and nuclear factor-kappa B (NF-κB) signalling in keratinocytes. During 2,4,6-trinitrobenzenesulfonic acid-induced colitis, the level of colonic myeloperoxidase (MPO) activity and the tissue levels of TNF-α, interleukin-1β (IL-1β) and IL-6 were drastically reduced by *Huangqin* decoction,a chinese therapeutic formula containing licorice as key candidate[Yang R,2017].

Glycyrrhiza glabra has been traditionally used to treat gastric ulcers, oral ulcers and ulcerative colitis. It has been shown to increase superoxide dismutase (SOD) enzymatic defence system significantly, besides reducing TNF-α, NO and IL-6 levels during acetic acid-induced ulcerative colitis [Zargari-Samadnejad A,2012].

1.5.1.1 Scientific Classification of *Glycyrrhiza Glabra*

Kingdom	:	Plantae – Plants
Subkingdom	:	Tracheobionta – Vascular plants
Superdivision	:	Spermatophyta – Seed plants
Division	:	Magnoliophyta – Flowering plants
Class	:	Magnoliopsida – Dicotyledons
Subclass	:	Rosidae

Order	:	Fabales
Family	:	Fabaceae – Pea family
Genus	:	*Glycyrrhiza* L. – licorice P
Species	:	*Glycyrrhiza glabra* L. – cultivated licorice P

Source:https://plants.usda.gov/java/ClassificationServlet?source=display&classid=Fabaceae

1.5.1.2 Availability of *Glycyrrhiza Glabra*

G. glabra is a herbaceous plant with a height of 1 m and consisting of 9-17 leaves, leaves are 7-15 cm in length, with bluish-white flowers and purple flowers from 0.8 to 1.2 cm in length. The fruits are oblong pods 2-3 cm long, containing several seeds with stolon roots. Licorice grows in fertile, clay or sandy soil, where water is available for the plant to grow. Roots are the most important medicinal parts of licorice that have been reported to be used alone or in combination with other herbs to treat many digestive disorders like stomach ulcers, excessive thirst, intestinal gas, and abdominal pain; respiratory tract disorders like coughs, asthma, tonsillitis, and sore throat; liver disorders like jaundice [Batiha GE,2020]. G. glabra is well documented to exhibit antibacterial, anti- inflammatory, antiviral, antioxidant, and antidiabetic activities [Pastorino G,2018].

1.5.1.3 Phytoconstituents of *Glycyrrhiza Glabra*

Phytochemical analysis of the plant root extracts showed that it majorly contains saponin triterpenes (glycyrrhizin, glycyrrhetinic acid and liquirtic acid) and flavonoids (liquirtin, isoflavonoids and formononetin). Not many investigations were done on the nourishing nature of G. glabra. But, liquorice is a wellspring of proteins, amino acids, polysaccharides and basic sugars, mineral salts (like calcium, phosphorus, sodium, potassium, iron, magnesium, silicon, selenium, manganese, zinc, and copper), gelatins, tars, starches, sterols, and gums The yellow shade of licorice is significantly due to the flavonoid content of the plant, which includes liquiritin and isoliquiritin [Kamei J,2003]. The essential oil derived from *G. glabra* is rich in propionic acid, benzoic acid, furfuraldehyde, 2,3- butanediol, furfuryl formate, maltol, 1- methyl- 2- formylpyrrole, and trimethylpyrazine. The triterpene saponins are the major constituents of licorice root, and are responsible for its characteristic sweetness.

1.6 Glycyrrhizin

The main water soluble and biologically active constituent of licorice root is glycyrrhizin(GZ). It is a triterpenoid saponin that is nearly multiple times sweeter than sucrose. GZ has been reported to have multiple therapeutic properties like immunomodulatory, anti-inflammatory, anti-ulcer, anti-allergic, antioxidant, anti-tumor, anti-diabetic, hepato and neuro protective. It is also used for the treatment of premenstrual syndrome and viral infections such as common cold, viral hepatitis, human immunodeficiency virus and acquired immunodeficiency syndrome [Li JY,2014]. GZ is presently of clinical interest for the treatment of chronic hepatitis. For instance, GZ has been used for more than 40 years in Japan, to treat liver diseases including chronic hepatitis, drug- or chemical-induced liver injury, nonalcoholic fatty liver disease, autoimmune hepatitis and hepatocellular carcinoma. It can be due to its inhibitory activity on inflammatory cytokines in the liver and activation of CD8+ T cells [Li X,2019]. GZ is known to modulate prime enzymes of various inflammatory pathways and oxidative stress. It downregulates many pro-inflammatory mediators TNF- α, IL-6, iNOS, and COX-2, thereby rendering protection against inflammation and ROS-induced damage [Maksoud HA,2019] [Gomaa AA ,2021].

The absorption, distribution, biotransformation and excretion of GZ and/or its monoammonium salts have been researched in rats and in human beings. The free form of GZ, or its monoammonium salt, is poorly absorbed from the gut. Inside the gastrointestinal tract, glycyrrhizinic acid is hydrolysed, primarily by the activity of intestinal microflora, to 18b-glycyrrhetic acid (the aglycone of glycyrrhizinic acid), a substance that gets readily absorbed. 18b-glycyrrhetic acid is subjected to enterohepatic circulation and can be further metabolized by intestinal bacteria to 3-dehydro-18b-glycyrrhetic acid and 3- epi-18b-glycyrrhetic acid. After absorbtion, glycyrrhetic acid is transported, primarily taken up into the liver by capacity-limited carriers, where it gets metabolized into glucuronide and sulfate conjugates and finally undergoes biliary excretion [Ploeger B,2001]. In brief, orally administered glycyrrhizin is totally hydrolyzed by intestinal bacteria and outreaches the systemic circulation as glycyrrhetinic acid.

1.6.1 Structural aspects of Glycyrrhizin

GZ is a triterpene saponin with a molecular formula $C_{42}H_{62}O_{16}$ and molecular weight 822.9 g/mol. Its IUPAC name is 6-[6-carboxy-2-[(11-carboxy-4,4,6a, 6b, 8a,11,14b-heptamethyl-14-oxo-2,3,4a,5,6,7,8,9,10,12,12a,14a-dodecahydro-1H-picen-3-yl)oxy]-4,5-dihydroxyoxan-3-yl]oxy-3,4,5-trihydroxyoxane-2-carboxylicacid) **(Figure 1.15)**. GZ is freely soluble in water and alcohol. Saponins are basically glycosides, which constitute one or more hydrophilic sugar chains attached to a hydrophobic backbone through glycosidic bonds, which can be a triterpene, a steroid alkaloid or a steroid. GZ has a hydrophobic aglycone 18β-glycyrrhetinic acid, attached to a di-glucuronic acid sugar chain through an ether bond [Ralla T,2020]. The well-known effect of GZ is pseudohyperaldosteronism, that can lead to elevated blood pressure. The joint FAO/WHO committee on evaluations on food additives, concluded that GZ is safe for consumption and an intake of 100 mg/day (about 2 mg/kg body weight per day) might not be causing adverse effects [Joint FA,2005].

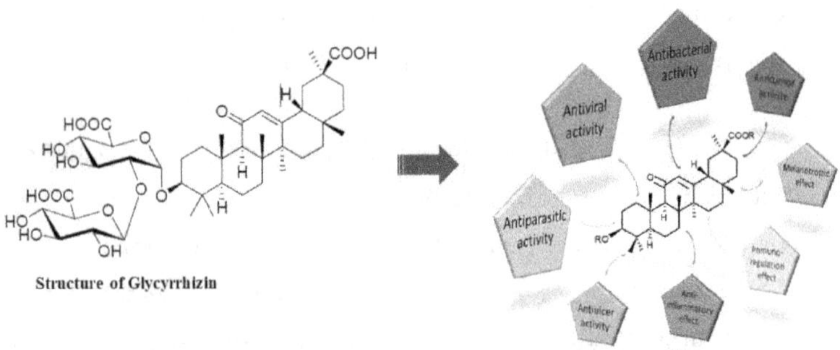

Figure 1.15 Chemical structure of glycyrrhizin and its pharmacological properties
(Source: https://sciendo.com/article/10.1515/cipms-2016-0024)

1.6.2 Glycyrrhizin- known pharmacological activities

High-mobility group box 1 protein (HMGB1) is a ubiquitous nuclear protein, but outside the cell it acts as a signaling protein of acute and chronic inflammation. HMGB1 is well-known biomarker of traumatic brain injury, neuroinflammation, epileptogenesis, cognitive dysfunctions and various other neurological diseases. GZ was shown to block HMGB1 secretion in the post ischemic brain by blocking its mitogenic and chemoattractant activities besides proinflammatory cytokine induction. Along with its neuroprotective effect, GZ was even shown to exhibit anti-oxidative effects in neurons [Kim SW,2012]. By seizing HMGB1, GZ ameliorates the production of inflammatory cytokines such as IL-18 and prevents contact dermatitis caused by contact allergens. As HMGB1 acts as a DAMPs, targeting HMGB1 is a very fruitful therapeutic approach in many cancers, inflammatory diseases and traumatic conditions.

Inflammation is a key complex biological response of body tissues, seen in many diseases like hepatitis, lung disease, Alzheimer's disease, rheumatoid arthritis, colonic inflammatory response, periodontitis etc. Stronger Neo-Minophagen C (SNMC, from Minophagen Pharmaceutical Co. Ltd., Tokyo) is a formulation of GZ, used for treating liver diseases in Japan for more than 40 years and broadly protects from a wide types of hepatic diseases like chronic viral hepatitis, drug- or chemical-induced liver injury, nonalcoholic fatty liver disease, autoimmune hepatitis and hepatocellular carcinoma [Li X,2019].

Recently, anti-coronavirus potential of GZ was investigated through docking studies. It has been shown that, it induces cholesterol-dependent disorganization of lipid rafts, essential for the cellular entry of corona virus, besides blocking HMGB1 and serum albumin. HMGB1 is very important for the viral infection and its pathogenicity. GZ was recorded to be good non-hemolytic saponin [Bailly C,2020]. It has already been well-researched against other viruses such as porcine epidemic diarrhea virus, its subsequent pro-inflammatory responses [Huan CC,2017] and varicella zoster virus [Baba M,1987]. The broad spectrum anti-viral, anti-bacterial, anti-inflammatory, anti-oxidative and immunomodulatory activities of licorice extract and its lead component GZ, along with their proposed mechanisms of action were provided comprehensively by Gomaa *etal.*, highlighting the rationale behind the presence of licorice and GZ in most traditional medicines [Gomaa AA ,2021]. Many clinical trials were registered on GZ, for its therapeutic effects on depression, Parkinson's disease, hepatocellular carcinoma, pancreatic cancer [Kwon YJ,2020] and recently for moderate COVID-19 pneumonia causing inflammation induced acute lung injury (ChiCTR2000029768 and ChiCTR2000030490) [Han R,2020].

2. REVIEW OF LITERATURE

2.1 Alcoholic CP

Chronic pancreatitis is an inflammatory phenomenon in pancreas, that progresses towards pancreatic parenchymal loss and fibrosis formation, ending up in pancreatic insufficiency and pancreatic damage. It occurs often in alcoholic men (70%) and sometimes with no known cause (30%) [JainD,2021]. Alcohol consumption larger than 5 drinks a day or >80 g/day in men and >50 g/day in women for several years, increases the risk of CP by 4-fold in a dose-dependent manner. One unit of alcohol is around 10 ml or 8 g of 100% ethanol. One drink is around 14 g of 100% ethanol or 1.75 units. An analysis with a total population of 146,517, that included 1671 persons with pancreatitis, showed a rapid dose-response relation between alcohol and the occurrence of pancreatitis [Irving HM,2009]. Disease spectrum of alcoholic CP is drastically increasing in India according to a prospective study conducted nationwide by Balakrishnan *etal.*, with 1086 subjects in 32 different centres [Balakrishnan V,2008]. Usually, CP is preceded by recurrent acute attacks and pain is the most common debilitating symptom. As per the data retrieved from a meta-analysis, in 10% of patients, CP occurred after a first episode of AP and in 36% of patients CP occurred after recurrent AP [Sankaran SJ,2015]. After an acute attack of pancreatitis around 50-80% of alcohol abusers develop CP. While, in many other cases, CP progresses quietly without any sort of acute episodes or pain, and clinical interest is mainly on treating the endocrine and exocrine insufficiencies [Hegyi P,2020]. Pancreatitis patients are advised to lead a healthy lifestyle, avoiding risk factors to avoid progression of AP to CP and pancreatic cancer. Pancreatic lipase and amylase stand as clinical means for the diagnosis of CP [Olesen SS,2019] [Klochkov A,2020].

Most of the detrimental effects of ethanol, are mediated by its toxic byproducts, acetaldehyde and FAEEs besides ROS. Acetaldehyde is shown to induce significant morphological changes in the rat and dog pancreas. It disturbs the stimulated secretory phenomenon of CCK [Majumdar AP,1986]. Acetaldehyde mainly depletes glutathione, which is an efficient cellular antioxidant to combat excessive ROS, whereas, oxidation of ethanol by CYP2E1 releases excess ROS. The imbalance leads to oxidative stress, a key pathological event in alcoholic CP. Oxidative stress destabilizes zymogen granules and lysosomes, thereby increasing the probability of intra-acinar activation of digestive enzymes [Apte MV,2003]. FAEEs are shown to accumulate in rat pancreas, cause acinar cell damage, lysosomal fragility, activation of trypsinogen and development of fibrotic changes [Haber PS,1993] [Lugea A,2003].

2.2 Cerulein

Cerulein, the analogue of CCK is documented to cause tremendous secretion of pancreatic enzymes like amylase and lipase, cytoplasmic vacuolization, death of acinar cells, edema formation, and inflammatory cell infiltration into the pancreas, as seen in human pancreatitis [Shen A,2017]. Cerulein is also reported to produce large amounts of ROS, activating NF-κB and thus causing cytokine expression in freshly isolated pancreatic acinar cells as explained by Yu etal.,[Yu JH,2002]. CCK receptors are G-protein-coupled receptors, which initiate transient $Ca2+$ oscillations by the activation of phospholipase C and induction of inositol triphosphate (IP3)-dependent $Ca2+$ release from pancreatic ER [Arnould M,2004] [Archer-Lahlou E,2005].

2.3 Alcohol and cerulein-induced CP

Many animal models have been recommended for the experimental induction of CP like ethanol feeding, repeated injections of cerulein or L-arginine, or injections of bile acids, oleic acid, or sodium taurocholate directly into the pancreatic duct, ligation of the common bile duct or pancreatic duct etc. Inclusion of ethanol to triggering factors like cerulein or L-arginine exacerbates pathologies of chronic pancreatitis like pancreatic fibrosis, inflammation, and acinar damage [Otsuki M,2010]. CP can be induced using frequent episodes of cerulein alone without ethanol, but pathological changes were recorded to be reversible. More specifically, cerulein-induced acinar injury is reversible [Obafemi TF,2018], whereas, chronic alcohol exposure at very high doses or as liquid diet or as continuous intragastric infusions did not result in a pronounced injury to the pancreas as documented earlier [Deng X,2005].

Compared to CP induction with either alcohol or cerulein alone, alcohol and cerulein mimicked various pathologies of CP, with respect to both etiology and physiology. It has been proved using IL-1β, TNF-α, TGF-β, α-SMA and myeloperoxidase activity as markers [Ahmadi A,2016]. During induction of CP using alcohol and cerulein, alcohol administration increases sensitivity of rats towards pancreatitis induced by repetitive Cer. The concerted action of alcohol and Cer lands up in activation of NF-kB and subsequent up-regulation of pancreatic pro-inflammatory cytokines and chemokines [Pandol SJ,1999].

2.4 Oxidative stress

Failure of cellular defensive mechanisms to combat ROS-induced damage, mitochondria in particular, leads to oxidative stress condition [Apte MV,2010]. During oxidative metabolism of ethanol, conversion to acetaldehyde by ADH and to acetate by ALDH, one molecule of NADH is produced in each reaction, supplying more reducing equivalents (NADH) to mitochondria as ALDH is a mitochondrial enzyme. Excess reducing equivalents facilitate transfer of electrons to molecular oxygen perpetuating the ROS generation. Alcohol is known to lower NAD+/NADH ratio in isolated acinar cells [Shalbueva N,2013]. So, ethanol exerts redox pressure in mitochondria through NADH, prompting the formation of ROS. Injury to the pancreas also causes a series of events like elevated ROS, inturn leading to oxidation of lipids, proteins and disruption of the pancreatic membrane. Oxidative stress is mostly accompanied by persistent inflammation, one of which is always induced by another. Oxidative stress plays critical role in the pathogenesis of various other chronic diseases like diabetes, cardiovascular and neurodegenerative diseases, alcoholic liver disease, and chronic kidney disease [Robles L,2013] [Biswas SK,2016].

A study by Meng *etal.*, demonstrated, the effect of the antioxidant resveratrol on NF-κB and inflammatory response in a rat model of pancreatitis. The resveratrol treated rats were shown to have significantly reduced levels of NF-κB, TNF-α, and IL-8 expressions compared to controls, besides reducing serum amylase, lipid peroxidation, intracellular calcium overload and myeloperoxidase in the pancreatitis rats. In addition, histological analysis of the pancreas showed lowered necrosis and edema [Meng Y,2005].

2.5 ER stress

Proper protein folding in the ER relies on optimal pH, calcium levels, oxidative conditions and availability of chaperones and enzymes like foldases and protein disulphide isomerases. ER stress is an early pathological event, documented in all models of experimental pancreatitis [Logsdon CD,2013]. Sensitive sensing and signaling mechanisms are evolved in pancreatic acinar cells and are known to be activated upon induction of ER stress. Moreover, ER stress has consequential effects in triggering inflammation and premature trypsinogen activation [Ren Z,2016]. Rats administered with alcoholic diet have evidenced an altered expression levels of several ER stress response genes like ATF3, a transcriptional regulator which mediates ATF4 pathway [Kubisch CH,2006]. An electron microscopy study demonstrated significant distention of the ER of pancreatic acinar cells and altered distribution of zymogen granules. Its experimental data in mice, even suggested alcohol feeding has a significant oxidative effect in the ER of the acinar cell besides increased expression of IRE1 and XBP1[Lugea A,2011]. Inside macrophages, CHOP is very crucial for the induction of caspase-11 mRNA and subsequent activation of pro-caspase-1 and the inflammasome [Endo M,2006].

Supramaximal doses of CCK-8 were reported to trigger all the UPR components like GRP78, PERK, XBP1, and CHOP expressions compared to submaximal doses of CCK-8 and other secretagogues like JMV-180 and bombesin in rat pancreatic acini [Kubisch CH,2007]. CHOP has a key role in progressing pancreatitis as previously reported by Suyama *et al.* [Suyama K,2008].

Signaling pathways regulating NFκB-mediated inflammatory responses, and the UPR were found to be connected with each other. Activated eIF2α of PERK pathway inhibits the translation of both NFκB and its inhibitor IκB, resulting in the activation of NFκB. And, the kinase function of IRE1 can phosphorylate IκB kinase (IKK) in response to stress, resulting in the degradation of IκBα and consequent NFκB activation [Hu P,2006].

Atrial natriuretic peptide has been shown to attenuate ER stress and favors ER-dependent apoptosis in cerulein-induced pancreatitis. Pretreatment with ANP reduced the expression of GRP78/Bip, which keeps the other stress sensor proteins inactive under non-stress states [Courreges AP,2019].

Protective effect of emodin on ER stress in rats, with sodium taurocholate induced pancreatitis was documented earlier. This study highlighted that the ER stress transducers Bip,

IRE1α, and their downstream molecules TRAF2, ASK1 were upregulated in pancreatitis. Furthermore, treatment with emodin reduced pancreatic injury by decreasing the release of amylase and inflammatory cytokines like TNF-α and IL-6. To conclude, emodin reduced pancreatic injury and prevented excess inflammatory reactions in pancreatitis, by inhibiting ER stress transducers [Wu L,2013].

2.6 Mitochondrial oxidative stress

ER and mitochondria are firmly interconnected physically and functionally through mitochondrial-associated membranes, which participates in Ca2+ signaling mechanisms [Bravo R,2012]. Excess ROS targets ER resident chaperones and ER Ca2+ channels(IP3R) leading to the release of Ca2+ from the ER into the cytosol inducing ER-stress signaling. The 7-ketocholesterol-activated UPR was shown to be suppressed by the antioxidant N-acetyl-cysteine in myocardial dysfunction [Guo R, 2009]. Similarly, polyphenols like curcumin and masoprocol act in neurodegenerative disorders [Pal R,2010], suggesting that this ER stress induction depends on oxidative stress.

ROS, physiologically produced as a consequence of ATP production in the mitochondria are important for cell signaling, also contribute to oxidative stress and subsequent cellular damage. Increased cytosolic calcium and calcium entry in mitochondria from ER can stimulate mitochondrial energy metabolism to produce more ROS by increasing the ubisemiquinone radical intermediate [St-Pierre J,2002]. Movement of calcium from the ER into the mitochondria induces stress signals and can activate opening of the MPTP, causing mitochondrial dysfunction and leading to the release of cytochrome c. The loss of cytochrome c inhibits respiratory complexes

[Grijalba MT,1999]. It has also been documented that, MPTP opening (triggered by $Ca2+$) causes few conformational changes in mitochondrial complex I, resulting in increased $H2O2$ production inhibition of complex I and increased of ROS production [Batandier C,2004].

The ETC complexes are not just the sole sources of ROS generation in mitochondria. α-ketoglutarate dehydrogenase complex (KGDHC) plays a crucial role in Ca2+-induced mitochondrial ROS production in addition to krebs cycle enzymes: isocitrate dehydrogenase and alpha-ketoglutarate dehydrogenase and pyruvate dehydrogenase. Excess mitochondrial Ca2+ stimulates Krebs cycle dehydrogenases, inturn increasing oxygen consumption and ROS production by increasing intra-mitochondrial NADH/NAD+ ratio [Tretter L,2004]. Mitochondrial Ca2+ also activates nitric oxide synthase, whose product NO·, disturbs the ETC complexes and enhances ROS generation. [Jekabsone A,2003]. Otherthan Ca2+-mediated mitochondrial ROS production, the ineffective cycles of disulfide bond formation and their breakage during ER stress might deplete cellular energy, stimulate mitochondrial respiration, and ultimately increase ROS production in mitochondria.

Excessively produced mitochondrial ROS also magnifies calcium flow from the ER into mitochondria in a positive feedback cycle. Decreased calcium concentrations in the ER lumen result in increased misfolding of proteins and activation of ER stress signalling pathways; as a whole, these actions can result in a vicious cycle of increased ER stress and ROS formation that leads to cellular damage. If there occurs an imbalance between ROS production and elimination, by either excessive production of ROS or impairment of the antioxidant defensive mechanisms, mitochondrial dysfunction occurs [Delierneux C,2020].

Increased ROS can also activate NF-κB and contribute directly to the development of local and systematic inflammation. NF-κB alters the transcription of a wide variety of genes, many of which promote inflammation like cytokines, chemokines and adhesion molecules.NF-κB has been considered as a target for new anti-inflammatory drugs. Early NF-kB activation is well reported to be associated with cerulein pancreatitis, and was shown to be activated in the pancreas within 30 min of cerulein infusion, when serum amylase and lipase levels just start to rise. Thus

NF-kB becomes activated in the pancreas at the onset of the disease itself. Furthermore, antioxidant N-acetylcysteine (NAC) was shown to block NF-kB activation, significantly improving parameters of pancreatitis by inhibiting intrapancreatic trypsin activation and mRNAexpression of cytokines like interleukin-6 [Gukovsky I,1998].

2.7 NLRP3 Inflammasome

Pancreatic acinar cell death releases DAMPs into the extracellular space triggering inflammation. Acinar cells and recruited inflammatory cells have pattern recognition receptors to recognise the released DAMPs. DAMPs mediate the assembly and activation of inflammasomes, which are the intracellular inflammatory multiprotein complexes, responsible for the activation of inflammatory responses. Signalling through pattern recognition receptors (PRR) like toll like receptor (TLR) 4 and 9 results in NF-κB facilitated inflammasome activation. NLRP3 is the specific inflammasome activated in pancreas in response to pancreatic cell injury. Activation of NLRP3 inflammasome causes the release of active caspase-1, a cytosolic protease which converts pro IL-1 beta and pro-IL-18 to active IL-1beta and IL-18 [Watanabe T, 2017].

Danger signals from mitochondria in response to stress also induces the formation of inflammasomes. Activation of inflammasomes by damaged mitochondria ends up in a caspase-1-dependent secretion of the inflammatory cytokines IL-1β and IL-18, often in the presence of NF-κB activation [Boaru SG,2015]. Interestingly, processing and releasing of IL-1β relies on the release of Ca2+ from intracellular ER stores as evidenced by a study on the Inhibition of IL-1β release by the membrane-permeable Ca2+ chelator, BAPTA-AM [Brough D,2003].

This fact brought to light that, NLRP3 inflammasome senses mitochondrial dysfunction and may be a reason, for the frequent association of mitochondrial damage with most of the inflammatory diseases. Increased ROS is a probable mechanism inducing NLRP3 inflammasome activation, besides lysosomal damage, potassium (K+) efflux, calcium (Ca2+) influx, and DAMPs released from damaged mitochondria as presented in **figure 2.1** [Zhou R,2011] [Pereira CA,2020].

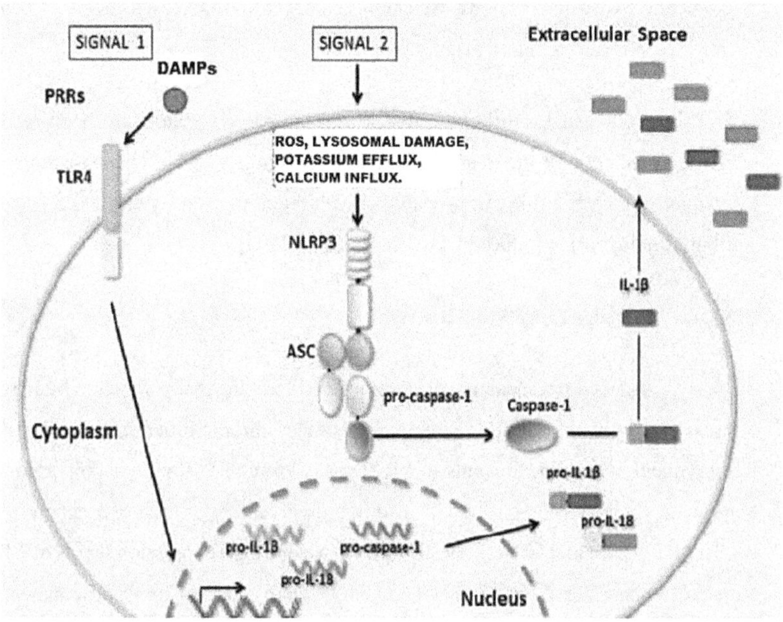

Figure 2.1 Activation of NLR3 inflammasome

(Source: https://www.tandfonline.com/doi/abs/10.3109/10409238.2012.694844?journalCode=ibmg20)

In a report on NLRP3 activation by *Chlamydia pneumoniae* lung infection, it has been illustrated clearly that, mitochondrial damage triggered induction of NLRP3-dependent IL-1β secretion in primed macrophages of a mouse model[Shimada K,2011].

In an another report, it has been shown that intra-articular administration of mitochondrial DNA, a DAMP extracted from human and murine tissues induced inflammatory arthritis in mice, and furthermore it is associated with increased TNF-α levels. This highlighted the association of mitochondrial DAMPs and inflammatory responses [Collins LV,2004].

2.8 Drugs for the treatment of CP

Bromhexine hydrochloride, a bronchial mucolytic, that when administered to 12 patients with alcoholic CP, shown to improve the symptoms of CP and pancreatic exocrine functions. An improvement in the increased levels of pancreatic enzymes was also reported [Tsujimoto T,2005].

Camostat mesilate (CM), an oral protease inhibitor, has been reported to be used clinically for the treatment of CP. Interestingly, CM has been demonstrated to attenuate pancreatic fibrosis, probably via inhibition of monocytes and PSC activity in dibutyltin dichloride induced CP in rats [Gibo J,2005].

2.8.1 Drugs targeting ER stress

It is very clear from the existing literature that, mitochondrial oxidative stress and activation of NF-κB and various other chronic inflammatory responses are subsequent pathological events to ER stress. Chronic ER stress was reported in mice pancreatic acinar cells during CP, with the involvement of high expression of ATF4, CHOP, GRP78, and XBP1 [Sah RP,2014]. A very high expression levels of ER stress marker genes like ATF6, XBP1 and CHOP were reported by Zhou etal., in human clinical specimens. According to this report, a humanized PRSS1 transgenic mouse was created and treated with cerulein to induce CP. Pathological alterations as observed were collagen deposition, and increased expression of the inflammatory factors IL-6, IL-1β, and TNF-α. ATF6, XBP1, and CHOP expression levels were also increased during CP development in this model [Zhou L,2019].

Many natural products are capable of interfering with ER stress, in a wide range of diseases like inflammatory diseases, cancers, lung diseases, neurodegenerative diseases and diabetes acting either as ER modulators or ER stress inducers or ER protectors [Martucciello S,2020].

Morusin, a flavonoid of root bark of Morus australis was able to induce ER stress by increasing the expression of GRP78/BiP, CHOP and IRE1α in human epithelial ovarian cancer. As a result, cells underwent paraptosis-like cell death, besides dilation of the ER and mitochondria, due to the release of Ca2+ from the ER to mitochondria [Xue J,2018]. A recent review highlighted the ability of natural compounds like curcumin, resveratrol, green tea polyphenols, quercetin, garcinia xanthones and benzophenones, and tocotrienols, to exert similar ER stress-related anticancer activity in different cancers [Limonta P,2019].

Induction of GRP78 and CHOP by indomethacin, as reported in gastric mucosal cells and human embryonic kidney cells (HEK293) was believed to be the mechanism of action behind apoptosis induced by NSAIDs, in fighting against cancer [Tsutsumi S,2004].

Thymoquinone, a monoterpene derivative of Nigella sativa seeds, has been reported to protect ischemia-reperfusion injury in liver by the attenuation of oxidative stress, mitochondrial damage, and ER stress and apoptosis. Resultant therapeutic effect was hypothesized to be brought, by the reduction of the expression of ER stress chaperones like GRP78 and CHOP, and caspase-12, because of its antioxidant nature. Additionally, thymoquinone inhibited apoptotis by decreasing cytochrome C release, besides decreasing caspase-9 and caspase-3 activition [Bouhlel A,2017].

ER stress activated in cerulein induced-AP, was reported to be significantly attenuated by tauroursodeoxycholic acid. TUDCA reduced the UPR genes like GRP78, pPERK, XBP-1, pJNK, CHOP; and caspase-12 and caspase-3 activation. It also inhibited ER stress-associated proapoptotic pathways. To conclude, TUDCA played a cytoprotective role in the exocrine pancreas [Seyhun E,2011]. Similarly, 4-phenylbutyric acid reduced the expression of ER stress markers like GRP78, CHOP, PERK, ATF 6, and IRE1 in vital organs (kidney, liver, lung, pancreas) of sodium taurocholate-induced AP rats besides significantly reducing apoptosis [Hong YP,2018].

Not just the pure compounds, the activity of natural extracts targeting ER stress were also reported in cancers. Trichosanthin, a traditional Chinese herb from the root tuber of Trichosanthes kirilowii, shown to have anticancer activities by inducing apoptosis in various cancer cell lines [Li J,2007].

ER stress may trigger inflammatory responses. Curcumin has been well documented to exhibit anti-inflammatory activities against bacterial infection, in Caco-2 and T84 intestinal epithelial cells causing downregulation of ER stress, as reported by decreased gene expression of GRP78, IRE1α and XBP1.Curcumin treatment targets ER stress and brings out its inflammatory response [Cho JA,2015].

2.8.2 Drugs targeting mitochondrial oxidative stress

Anetholtrithion (OP2113) is an antioxidant, commonly recommended for salivary secretion in conditions of dry mouth, as an adjunctive for cholecystitis, gallstones, indigestion, and hepatitis. It has been reported to decrease ROS production in isolated rat heart mitochondria, by not just acting as free radical scavenger but by directly and specifically inhibiting ROS production, at the site IQ (quinone site) of mitochondrial complex I of ETC. It may be implicated in various disorders like aging, Parkinson's, Alzheimer's diseases, cardiac atrial fibrillation, and ischemia-reperfusion injury, in which ROS-induced mitochondrial dysfunction occurs [Detaille D,2019].

A report on Mito Q, a mitochondria-targeted antioxidant revealed that, Mito Q challenged H2O2-induced intracellular ROS production in murine pancreatic acinar cells. It has been reported to decrease pancreatic MPO activity, reduced ROS production in PMN leukocytes by targeting NADPH oxidase, highlighting the ROS scavenging property of MitoQ but with no significant improvements in pancreatic histopathology [Huang W,2015]. SkQ1, an another studied mitochondria-targeted antioxidant, has been shown to quench ROS more effectively in CP, as its antioxidant activity was reported to be exhibited even at nM concentrations besides having a significant effect in decreasing pain-associated behavior in rats [Weniger M,2016].

2.9 Natural products for the treatment of CP

Gardenia jasminoides (GJ) was reported to hold a pancreato-protective effect against cerulein-induced CP. Its aqueous extract elicited anti-inflammation and antifibrotic effects by inhibiting c-Jun N-terminal kinase (JNK) and extracellular signal-regulated protein kinase (ERK) activation during CP. Furthermore, GJ reduced pancreatic edema and inflammatory cell infiltration [Choi JW,2020].

Piperine, a natural alkaloid of black pepper, has been reported to exhibit anti-inflammatory, anti-oxidative, and pancreato-protective effects. Piperine treatment decreased the expression of fibrosis mediators, like α-smooth muscle actin (α-SMA), collagen, and fibronectin 1 in the pancreas and PSCs. Besides, it reduced the production of transforming growth factor (TGF)-β in the pancreas and PSCs [Lee SK,2019].

Nardostachys jatamansi (NJ), a widely used gastrointestinal remedy drug for inflammation, was shown to ameliorate ACP by inhibition of PSC activation and collagen deposition [Bae GS,2012].

Few polyphenols with anti-inflammatory characteristics like resveratrol, epigallocatechin gallate, curcumin, and quercetin were reported to alleviate the symptoms of pancreatitis. Ingestion or systemic administration of these agents has been shown to inhibit various NFκB - dependent gene expressions [Shapiro H,2007].

A cross-sectional survey conducted at a pancreatic disorders outpatient clinic, over a 6-month time frame reported that, 45% of the pancreatitis patients relies on alternative medicines. Artemisinin, Curcumin, Emodin, Hesperidin, Naringin, Rutin, Resveratrol, Rhein were the reported effective phytochemicals with proven mechanism of action against pancreatitis[Gaman L,2018]. In a recent Ayurvedic study where CP is termed as Tikshnoshna pitta, Guduchi (*Tinospora cordifolia* Willd. Miers.ExHook.), Yashtimadhu (*Glycyrrhiza glabra* Linn.), a salt preparation Narikela lavana and Sutashekhara rasa (without gold) have been formulated to treat CP. 2g of guduchi, 2g of yashtimadhu, 0.5g of narikelalavana and 0.5g sutashekhara rasa without gold, has been prescribed to every patient two times a day for 2 months. According to the report, pain has been reduced by 90.25%, nausea and vomiting reduced by 62.5%, flatulence reduced by 48.05%. Additionally, increased serum amylases and lipases were found to be restored significantly, in 28 established cases after this treatment. And no such adverse effects noted [PradyotBikashKar,2017].

2.9.1 *Glycyrrhiza glabra* –in classical texts

Ayurvedic name	:	Yashtimadhu
Siddha name	:	Athimadhuram
Unani name	:	Asl-us-soos, Rubb-us-soos (Extract)
English name	:	Licorice/ Liquorice
Part used	:	Root
Dose	:	3-5g

2.9.1.1 Uses documented in Ayurveda

- ✓ More than 17 medicinal oils are contained in the drug and were used for epilepsy, paralysis, rheumatism, haemorrhagic diseases.
- ✓ In edema, the paste of yashtimadhu, Tila (*Sesamum Indicum*) and milk mixed with butter, was suggested.
- ✓ Its decoction was applied on erysipelas, a bacterial infection as documented in Charaka samhitaa, Sushruta samhitaa, Vrindamaadhava, which are comprehensive texts on ancient Indian medicine.
- ✓ After surgery, clarified butter mixed with yashtimadhu was prescribed as external application for haemorrhoids as recorded in Sushruta samhitaa.
- ✓ Yashtimadhu churna is available for cough, bronchitis, hoarness of voice.
- ✓ Yashtyaadi Kashaya is suggested for diarrhea with blood and menorrhagia.
- ✓ Nilibringaadi taila, Duurvadi taila, Balaashwaganda-laakshaadi taila, Asanvilvaadi taila prescribed for hair and skin problems, has yashtimadhu as a key ingredient.
- ✓ It is a major component in Naarikelannjana eyedrops recommended for conjunctivitis. [Nadkarni KM. Indian materia medica,1996]

2.9.1.2 Uses documented in Unani

- ✓ Asl-us-soos *(Glycyrrhiza glabra)* is a major ingredient in Habb-e-shaheeqa prescribed for migrane and dry cough; Laooq-e-Nazli given for bronchitis; Laooq-e-zeeq-un-nafas for brochial asthma and catarrhal inflammation of nasal mucus membrane.
- ✓ Marham-e-jadwar given for ulcers, lymphadenitis [Salim S,2018].

2.9.1.3 Uses documented in other cultures

- ✓ Oral licorice preparations are recommended for the treatment of viral infections like common cold, viral hepatitis, HIV, AIDS, premenstrual syndrome, inflammations, ulcerative conditions of GIT and as topical preparations for eczema, herpes, psoriasis in the native cultures of west regions.

- ✓ Glycyrrhiza root was an effective Kampo (traditional Japanese medicine) herb, found efficient for treatment of glossodynia, the burning mouth syndrome.

- ✓ G. glabra was listed in plants with reported immunomodulatory properties, in traditional Iranian medicine.

- ✓ Licorice was the key component in traditional Chinese medicinal formulas, used in treating helicobacter pylori-related gastropathy, inflammatory bowel syndrome and Tai yang diseases (diseases of the exterior, like common cold).

- ✓ It was among the top medicinal plants highly recommended in traditional Persian medical texts for the treatment of asthma.

- ✓ German commission E monograph recognized *Glycyrrhiza glabra* herb's efficacy especially for the treatment of cough, bronchitis and gastritis. Additionally, it is the most culturally important taxa as documented by American botanical council, an herbal library.

https://www.herbalgram.org/resources/herbmedpro/herb-list/glycyrrhiza-glabra-g-uralensis/

2.10 Anti-inflammatory actions of Glycyrrhizin

Glycyrrhizin is basically composed of an aglycone called 18β-glycyrrhetinic acid (GE), that is a pentacyclic triterpene derivative of the β-amyrin type, a D-glucuronic acid dimer which is linked to the aglycone through a glycosidic bond as represented in **figure 2.2**.

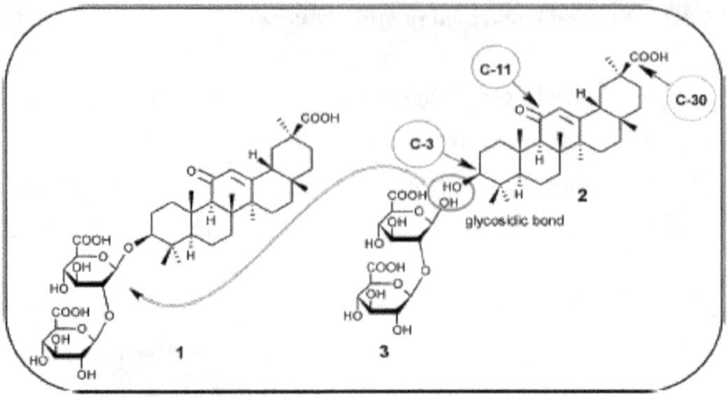

Figure 2.2 Pentacyclic triterpene system of GZ

(Source: https://sciendo.com/article/10.1515/cipms-2016-0024)

During inflammatory responses in AP, many chemokines gets released from leukocytes and pancreatic acinar cells, playing a key role in pancreatic pathophysiology. Among them, monocyte chemoattractant protein-1 (MCP-1 or CCL2) and macrophage inhibitory protein-2 (MIP-2 or CXCL2) are very important and have been reported to be elevated in the plasma of patients with AP. Panahi *etal*., demonstrated that glycyrrhizin (GZ) ameliorated AP, by downregulating the expression of CXCL2 and CCL2 at mRNA levels in the isolated pancreatic acinar cells, in experimental rats induced AP [Panahi Y,2015]. It has also been reported that, GZ attenuates neutrophil and monocytes accumulation in pancreas, reducing pancreatic tissue injury and underlying inflammatory responses in AP [Fakhari S,2014].

Glycyrrhizin was reported to reduce the levels of pro-inflammatory cytokines and downregulate the expression of HMGB1, besides improving the congestion, edema, disorganization of pancreatic lobules and pancreatic lesions in mice with AP [Pan YL,2014].

It is a very good example for a compound with effective structure active relationship. By introducing a variety of functional groups, or by modifying the GE pentacyclic triterpene skeleton, particularly at C-3, C-11 and C-30, many compounds of different pharmacological value can be made, with potent anti-ulcer, anti-inflammatory, hepatoprotective, antimicrobial, antiparasitic and antiviral properties [Langer D,2016].

3. SCOPE OF THE STUDY

Chronic pancreatitis, characterized by persistent inflammation in pancreas causes progressive and significant damage to the glandular organ. This results in exocrine and endocrine pancreatic insufficiency that leads to severe abdominal pain, maldigestion, malnutrition and weight loss. Globally, around 16,45,000 people are known to be affected with this gastrointestinal disorder. In India, the incidence keeps increasing every year mainly due to alcohol abuse. The major risk factor of CP in India is studied to be the overconsumption of alcohol.

The key cells present in pancreas, which produce digestive enzymes contain abundant endoplasmic reticulum to mete out the highest rate of protein synthesis. This multifunctional organelle also stores calcium, apart from having major responsibility of proper protein folding and processing to remove unwanted peptide fragments of a peptide protein. When these misfolded proteins accumulate in ER, it exerts stress in the organelle with the activation of a specific stress response pathway, the unfolded protein response(UPR) and it is shown to be influenced by alcohol derived metabolites such as acetaldehyde, fatty acid ethyl esters and also lipid peroxidation products (ROS).

The resultant elevation in ROS production in the cell is reflected also in mitochondrial function through the mobilization of calcium from ER to mitochondria. Also, during ER stress the accumulated unfolded proteins elicits Ca2+ leakage to mitochondria. The oxidative stress in mitochondria results in the deficient mitochondrial functions mainly electron transport process. Among the five ETC complexes, any one or more have been shown to be disturbed in pathological conditions. In this event, mitochondrial morphology is disturbed and may lead to shedding of damaged components, which can act as damage associated molecular patterns (DAMPs) and trigger the multi-protein complex known as inflammasomes. Inflammasomes are induced in any organ when the cells are insulted with proinflammatory agents, just to protect the organ from damage merely by producing anti inflamamtory cytokines. But this triggering event, if occurs in an uncontrolled manner, cytokines are produced in large amount and may lead to inflammation and cellular injury.

Many allopathic medicines have been recommended to alleviate the symptoms of CP and even to heal the injured portion of the organ. But, not even a single drug is fully recommended to give a complete cure. From ancient times, traditional system of medicine i.e. ayurvedic system of medicine is in common practice for major human ailments. In India, the plant based medicines are vast in use due to less cost, easy availability and less side effects. In this regard, it is considered essential to invent new herbal drugs to combat the ill-effects of CP. Since as it is explained earlier, ER stress, oxidative stress and mitochondrial factors are involved in the pathogenesis of CP, any drug to be invented for CP need to be tested whether the drugs of interest can target these factors and thereby, a novel pathway can be generated and the drug can be scientifically validated.

In this regard, Glycyrrhiza *glabra* root extract and the major component Glycyrrhizin were tested in experimental rats administered with alcohol and cerulein, that mimics human CP. Since 70% aqueous alcohol extract has almost all the phytonutrients including saponins, this extract (HAELR) was used for the study.

The present study is aimed

- To identify and quantify the major phytoconstituents present in HAELR
- To assess the acute toxicity profile, LD_{50} value and chronic toxicity profile of HAELR and glycyrrhizin.
- To find out the optimal dose of HAELR and glycyrrhizin for further efficacy study.
- To check whether ER stress response activated in CP can be attenuated by HAELR/ glycyrrhizin co-administration by analyzing the expression of markers of UPR and ER stress factors like ATF4, CHOP, GRP78, XBP1.
- To check whether HAELR/glycyrrhizin co-administration preserves the antioxidant status in pancreatic mitochondria to give protection against mitochondrial oxidative stress at the site of origin itself.

- To check whether mitochondrial calcium overload and mitochondrial dysfunction be augmented by HAELR /glycyrrhizin co-administration.

- To determine the antioxidant potential of HAELR/glycyrrhizin co-administration against cellular oxidative stress caused by ethanol and cerulein administrations.

- To study the effect of HAELR/glycyrrhizin co-administration on the expression levels of NF-κB, an inducible transcription factor of inflammatory response and a central mediator for activating cytokines and chemokines.

- To investigate the effect of HAELR/glycyrrhizin co-administration on the components of NLRP3 inflammasome such as caspase-1 and the cytokines like IL-1β and IL-18 which are highly involved in pancreatic cell damage and progression of pancreatitis.

- To check whether glycyrrhizin has binding affinity towards UPR components- GRP78 and ATF4 by *in silico* study.

The outcome of the study is expected to scientifically validate Glycyrrhiza glabra root extract and Glycyrrhizin as the drugs for CP, throwing more light on the novel anti-inflammatory effect of the test drugs in terms of ER stress and mitochondrial dysfunction.

4. MATERIALS AND METHODS

4.1 Chemicals and reagents

Glycyrrhizin was obtained from TCI chemicals, Chennai, India. Cerulein (C9026-1MG) was purchased from Biovision, California, USA. Amylase (AMY DS:01P) and lipase (LIP UV:01P) assay kits were from Pure Chemicals Co, Chennai, India. IL-1β (ab100767) and caspase-1(ab39470) kits were procured from Merckmillipore, Massachusetts, United States. IL-18 (KRC2341) kit was from Thermo Fisher scientific, Mumbai, India. RNeasy Miniprep kit and DNase I (Catalogue#M0303S) were purchased from Quaigen, Hilden, Germany and New england biolabs, Massachusetts, USA, respectively. cDNA reverse transcription kit (Catalogue#4368814) was purchased from Applied biosystems, California, USA. RNA later (Cat. #R0901) was obtained from Sigma- Aldrich, Saint Louis, MO. Fura-2AM was from Merck, Mumbai, India. Mitochondrial complex-1 activity microplate assay kit (ab109721) was obtained from Abcam, Cambridge, MA.

4.2 Glycyrrhizin preparation

Glycyrrhizin is freely soluble in water and no specific preparation is needed.

4.3 Plant collection and identification

The roots of licorice were purchased from local drug stores of chennai. The roots were verified and certified (No#2016-3303) by Prof. P. Jayaraman, a renowned plant taxonomist in Chennai.

4.4 Preparation of hydroalcoholic extract of licorice root (HAELR)

The roots of *Glycyrrhiza glabra* were surface cleaned, shade-dried, pulverized and macerated with 70% aqueous ethanol at room temperature (RT) for 48 hours by frequently agitating in a shaker [Handa SS,2008]. The mixture obtained was strained, soaked again in ethanol. This process of maceration was repeated three to four times. The extract was filtered using Whatmann no.1 filter paper, evaporated to dryness and lyophilized to obtain a homogenous residue, which was stored at 4 °C. The extract was stored in sterile vials in portions until analyses. The yield was found to be 12% w/w.

4.5 Qualitative and Quantitative analysis of HAELR

4.5.1 High performance liquid chromatography (HPLC) analysis of HAELR

HPLC analysis was carried out on Shimadzu HPLC CLASS-VPTM series equipped with 2489 UV/Visible detector for the identification and quantification of phytochemicals in HAELR. EZ Chrom Elite Data System was used for data acquisition, processing, controlling of HPLC and reporting data.

4.5.1.1 Identification and quantification of flavonoids

About 10 g of HAELR was refluxed with the extraction solvent - alcohol, water and hydrochloric acid mixture (50:20:8) - on a hot water bath for 135 min to hydrolyse glycosides to aglycones, followed by decantation and sonication for 30 min using methanol. The contents were filtered and diluted to 100 mL with methanol. The reference standards used were quercetin, kaempferol, isorhamnetin, galangin, luteolin, rutin and thymoquinone. Methanol-water-phosphoric acid (100:100:1) was the mobile phase. Waters symmetry C-18-column with a flow rate of 1.5 mL per minute was used. Isocratically eluted compounds were detected by UV detector at 270 nm. The flavonoids were identified and quantified using their retention times, and comparing with that of standards.

4.5.1.2 Identification and quantification of saponins

Equal volumes of glycyrrhizin standard and sample (20 μL) were separately injected into the chromatograph and the separation was carried out by isocratic elution. Methanol-water-acetic acid mixture (60:34:6) was the mobile phase used. The flow rate was 1 mL/min through a C-18- reverse phase column. Measurement of UV absorbance was done at 254 nm. Saponins were identified and quantified in HAELR using their retention times and comparing with that of standards.

4.5.2 Gas chromatography coupled to mass spectrometry (GC-MS) analysis of HAELR

HAELR was subjected to gas chromatography analysis on Agilent-N6890series gas chromatograph with an analytical column (19091J-413). It is coupled to a mass spectrometer (JEOL- GC-MATE-II), at a voltage of 70 eV. The mass spectral scan range of the mass analyser was set to 50-600 amu. Carrier gas used was helium, at a constant flow rate of 1 mL/min. The GC-oven was set at a ramp rate from 50 °C -250 °C at 10 °C /min. Compounds were identified using NIST-database.

4.6 Experimental animals

Male albino Wistar rats weighing 175-200 g were maintained on a 12-hour light-dark cycle at 25°C, humidity between 60% and 70%. The rats were housed in polyethylene cages, and given free access to standard rat chow pellet diet and water during the acclimatization period. Institutional Animal Ethics Committee approved the experimental protocol. (XIX/VELS/PCOL/06/2000/CPCSEA/IAEC/03.10.2016) (XXIII/VELS/PCOL/01/2000/CPCSEA/ IAEC / 07.02.2020)

4.7 Toxicity studies

4.7.1 Toxicity Estimation Software Tool (TEST)

The Toxicity Estimation Software Tool (TEST) is used for the assessment of toxicity of glycyrrhizin. TEST calculates the toxicity using a variety of Quantitative Structure Activity Relationship (QSAR) methodologies. The structure of glycyrrhizin is imported from PDB database that serves as an input in TEST. Once entered, the toxicity is automatically calculated using one of QSAR methodologies by TEST.

4.7.2 Acute toxicity study

Acute toxicity study was conducted according to the OECD guidelines (Test: 423). Rats were divided into 6 groups (where "n" is six) and the animal arrangement is as follows. Rats were administered with HAELR, orally prior to food till 14days.

STUDY GROUPS

GROUP I - Control, given standard pellet diet and water *ad libitum.*

GROUP II - In addition, rats were administered 500mg/kg b.wt. of HAELR orally.

GROUP III - In addition, rats were administered 1000mg/kg b.wt. of HAELR orally.

GROUP IV - In addition, rats were administered 2000mg/kg b.wt. of HAELR orally.

GROUP V - In addition, rats were administered 4000mg/kg b.wt. of HAELR orally.

GROUP VI - In addition, rats were administered 5000mg/kg b.wt. of HAELR orally.

In this acute toxicology testing, the drug was administered as single dose in the morning before food by leaving rats fasted overnight and effect of the drug was observed for 14 days. Mortalities caused by the drug during the experimental period were recorded. The animals were also observed for their level of food and water intake, weight loss, tremors, convulsions, salivation, diarrhea, lethargy, decreased locomotion and its duration every one hour for the first 24 hours and then for 14days. Any mortality during the exposure was noted.

After 14days, rats were sedated using diethylether and sacrificed by manual neck dislocation. Blood was drawn, serum separated and the biochemical and hematological parameters for toxicity profile were assessed. Vital organs like liver, kidney, heart, pancreas and brain were excised for histopathological studies. LD_{50} was calculated according to arithmetical method of Karber [Turner R,2013].

4.7.3 Chronic toxicity study

Rats were divided into 6 groups (where "n" is six) and the arrangement is as follows. Rats were administered with HAELR, orally prior to food till 90days.

Group I -Control, given standard pellet diet and water *ad libitum.*

Group II - In addition, rats were administered 50mg/kg b.wt. of HAELR orally.

Group III - In addition, rats were administered 100mg/kg b.wt. of HAELR orally.

Group IV - In addition, rats were administered 200mg/kg b.wt. of HAELR orally.

Group V - In addition, rats were administered 400mg/kg b.wt. of HAELR orally.

Group VI - In addition, rats were administered 500mg/kg b.wt. of HAELR orally.

After 90days, rats were sedated by diethylether and euthanised by manual neck dislocation. Blood was drawn, serum separated and the biochemical and hematological parameters for toxicity profile were assessed. Vital organs like liver, kidney, heart, pancreas and brain were excised for histopathological studies.

4.7.4 Biochemical analysis to test the toxicity profile of HAELR.

Assay of AST, ALT, ALP, LDH; estimation of urea, creatinine, glucose and protein; and determination of antioxidants GSH, GPx, SOD and CAT were carried out in blood samples.

4.7.4.1 Assay of aspartate transaminase (AST) and alanine transaminase (ALT)

AST&ALT assay→ **King(1965a)**.

Reagents required

1. Phosphate buffer (100 mM, pH 7.4).
2. Substrate for AST→ 2.66g of aspartate & 38mg of 2-oxoglutarate were weighed separately and dissolved in a small volume of prepared buffer initially, by warming up a little. Final volume of substrate was made to 100 ml with the same buffer.
3. Substrate for ALT→ 1.78g of alanine & 38mg of 2-oxoglutarate were weighed separately and dissolved in the prepared buffer. 0.5ml of sodium hydroxide (1N) was added to enhance the solubility. Final volume was made to 100ml with the same buffer.

4. 2, 4-DNPH (1 mM in 2N HCl).

5. NaOH (0.4N).

6. Standard solution→ 110 mg of C3H3NaO3 in 100 ml of phosphate buffer was the standard. Suitably diluted working standard has a concentration of 1 μM pyruvate/ml.

This assay was conducted in serum samples

Experimental procedure

A volume of 1ml of respective substrates for AST and ALT, were taken in tests T1&T2 and in their corresponding controls C1&C2. All these test tubes were initially kept at RT for 5min. Serum (0.1ml) was then added to T1&T2 only. Both T1&T2 and C1& C2 were then incubated at RT, for 60min in case of AST and 30min in case of ALT. DNPH (1ml) was then added to stop the chemical-reaction. Serum(0.1ml) was added to C1 &C2 and incubated at RT for 10min. 0.4N sodium hydroxide (10 ml) was then added to all the tubes and the colour was read at 525 nm. A series of concentrations were made with sodium pyruvate standard using buffered substrates, treated likewise and the colour intensity was measured at 525 nm. Calculations were done through a calibration curve.

Result

Results were expressed as U/L.

4.7.4.2 Alkaline phosphatase (ALP) assay

ALP assay→ **Bowers &McComb (1975)**.

Reagents required

1. Assay-buffer → Aminomethylpropanol (84M dissolved in 15% HCl, pH 10.09).

2. $MgCl_2$ 1.5mM.

3. Substrate→ p-Nitrophenyl phosphate (215mM dissolved in 1.5mM $MgCl_2$).

This assay was conducted in serum samples

Experimental procedure

Buffer(2.8ml) and serum(0.1ml) were mixed with each other, kept at RT for 5 min. The chemical reaction was made to start with 0.2ml substrate. Buffer stands as the reference in the assay. Change in absorbance was recorded at 450nm at an interval of 30 seconds for 5 min in spectrophotometer.

Result

Results were expressed as U/L.

4.7.4.3 Lactate dehydrogenase (LDH) assay

LDH assay→ **King(1965b)**.

Reagents required

1. Assay-buffer → 0.1 M glycine (7.5 g) and NaCl (5.85 mg) were dissolved in 1000ml of distilled water (DH2O).
2. NaOH (0.1N)
3. NaOH (0.4N)
4. HCl (2N)
5. Substrate→ Lithium lactate (2.78 g) was made to dissolve slowly in 125 ml of glycine buffer with the simultaneous addition of NaOH (0.1N, 75 ml) solution. This was made fresh.
6. NAD+ solution→ NAD+ (5mg) was mixed in DH2O (1ml) just before use.

7. Dinitrophenylhydrazine→ 20 mg of DNPH was dissolved in 100ml of 2N hydrochloric acid just before use.

8. C3H3NaO3 solution→ C3H3NaO3(11 mg) was taken in 100ml of buffer.

   Concentration = 1μM/ml

This assay was conducted in serum samples

Experimental procedure

Substrate of 1ml volume and enzyme source of 0.1ml volume were added to each other and kept at RT for 15 min. To this, 0.2 ml of NAD+ solution was added and incubation was proceeded for 15 min. DNPH reagent (1ml) was added subsequently to stop the chemical reaction and incubated for further 15 minutes at RT. To this, 7ml of 0.4N NaOH was added. Brown colour obtained was read at 420 nm in spectrophotometer.

Result

Results were expressed as U/L.

4.7.4.4 Estimation of Urea

Estimation of urea →**Natelson(1951).**

Reagents required

1. Working standard solution→ 10mg of urea in 100ml DH2O.

Concentration = 100 μg/ml

2. Na2WO4→10%

3. H_2 SO_4 →0.07N

4. DAM (Diacetylmonoxime)→ DAM (2g) was dissolved in 2% CH_3 COOH

5. Mixture of H3PO4& H_2SO_4 →25ml of concentrated H_2SO_4 was slowly mixed with 75ml of 85% H3PO4 in an ice bath.

This assay was conducted in serum samples

Experimental procedure

To 0.1ml of serum-sample, 3.3ml of DH2O, 0.3ml of 10% Na2WO4 and 0.3ml of 0.07N H_2SO_4 were added, followed by centrifugation. To 1ml of resultant supernatant,1ml of DH2O, 0.4ml of DAM and 2.6ml of H3PO4&H_2SO_4 reagent were added and boiled for 30 min. Once cooled, OD was read at 480nm. Aliquots of standard urea were also processed likewise.

Results

Results were expressed as mg/dl

4.7.4.5 Estimation of Creatinine

Estimation of creatinine → **Slot (1965**).

Reagents required

1. Na2WO4→ 5%
2. H_2SO_4 → 2/3N
3. C6H3N3O7→ 0.04M
4. NaOH→ 0.75M
5. C2HCl3O2 → 10%
6. Stock standard: 100mg of creatinine in 100ml of 0.1N HCl

Concentration = 1mg/ml

7. Working standard: 1ml of the stock standard was made to 100ml with DH2O

This assay was conducted in serum samples

Sample processing

0.1ml serum sample and 3.9ml TCA (10%) were added to each other, followed by centrifugation. The resultant-supernatant was then estimated.

Experimental procedure

Aliquots of working standard (0.5-2.5ml) with various concentrations (5-25μg) were taken. 0.5ml of supernatant was taken separately. Volumes were made up to 8ml by DH2O and 8ml of DH2O itself was used as blank. 1ml of 0.75M NaOH and 1ml of 0.04M C6H3N3O7 were added to each, mixed and left to stay for 45 min. Brown colour formed was read at 520nm.

Result

Results were expressed as mg/dl.

4.7.4.6 Estimation of glucose

Estimation of glucose → **Godkar (1994)**

Reagents required

1. C14H16N2 reagent: 60ml of C14H16N2 and 1.5g of CH4N2S were mixed with each other, along with 940ml of CH_3 COOH.

2. TCA (10%).

3. Glucose standard: 10mg of glucose in 50ml of DH2O served as the standard. To this 30ml of 10% TCA was added, and the contents were made up to 100ml with DH2O.

   Concentration = 0.1mg/ml

This assay was conducted in whole blood samples

Sample processing

A volume of 0.5ml whole blood, 3ml DH2O and 1.5ml 10% TCA were added, mixed and allowed to stand for 10minutes and filtered. Thus the blood was made protein free.

Experimental procedure

A series of standards of glucose(0.2-1ml) were prepared for the estimation. 1ml of protein-free-filterate was also taken separately. 4ml of C14H16N2-reagent was added to each tube, mixed completely and boiled in water-bath for 10min. A blue-green colour formed was read at 620nm.

Results

Results were expressed as mg/dL

4.7.4.7 Estimation of protein

Estimation of protein → Bradford (1976).

Reagents required

1. PBS→ pH 7.4
2. Standard BSA→ 10mg BSA in 100ml PBS.

   Concentration = 100μg/ml

3. CBB dye→ CBB G250 (100mg) was taken in 95% C2H5OH (50ml) and 85% H3PO4 (100ml) and the entire volume was diluted to 1000ml with DH2O.

This assay was conducted in serum and tissue homogenate samples

Experimental procedure

Suitably diluted samples were made-up to 1ml using DH2O. 5ml of Bradford reagent was then added and mixed. From this mixture, 1ml was taken and diluted again with 4ml of DH2O followed by incubation for 30min. BSA-standards were prepared likewise and the absorbance was measured at 595nm and the concentration of protein was calculated.

Results

Results were expressed as g/dl in serum.

Serum levels of GSH and enzymatic antioxidants like GPx, SOD and CAT were determined in all the experimental rats subjected to acute and chronic oral exposure to HAELR, to assess oxidative stress after exposure to the drug (Methods in section 4.10.1.2).

4.7.5 Hematological analysis to test the toxicity profile of HAELR.

KX21N cell counter from sysmex, which can detect upto sixty samples an hour was utilized for the determination of hematological parameters. Hemoglobin, red blood cell count (RBC), white blood cell count(WBC) and platelet count were analysed to assess the toxic effect of HAELR.

This assay was conducted in whole blood in EDTA.

Results

Red blood cell, white blood cell and platelet counts were expressed as-million per mm^3, cells per mm^3 and lakhs per mm^3, respectively, whereas hemoglobin was expressed as g%.

4.8 Alcohol& cerulein-induced chronic pancreatitis

Male Wistar rats were administered alcohol (0%-36% of total calories for 5 weeks) and cerulein (20 μg/kg b.wt i.p, three times a week for last three weeks) to induce chronic pancreatitis.

4.9 Dose response study

Rats were sorted into six groups, where "n" is six.

STUDY GROUPS

Group I Control, standard pellet diet and water *ad libitum*.

Group II Rats were given alcohol and cerulein.

Group III In addition, rats were coadministered 25mg/kg bodyweight of HAELR orally.

Group IV In addition, rats were coadministered 50mg/kg bodyweight of HAELR orally.

Group V In addition, rats were coadministered 100mg/kg bodyweight of HAELR orally.

Group VI In addition, rats were coadministered 200mg/kg bodyweight of HAELR orally.

After 5weeks, rats were sedated by diethylether and euthanised by manual neck dislocation. Blood was drawn and immediately the serum was separated. Estimation of lipase, amylase, myeloperoxidase, caspase-1, IL-1β and IL-18 in fresh serum was conducted.

4.10 Therapeutic efficacy of HAELR and GZ

STUDY GROUPS

I- Group: Control	Standard pellet diet and water *ad libitum* for the total experimental period of 5weeks
II- Group: HAELR control	Normal diet for first 2weeks and 100mg/kg b.wt of HAELR for last 3weeks
III- Group: GZ control	Normal diet for first 2weeks and 10mg/kg b.wt of glycyrrhizin for last 3weeks
IV- Group: Ethanol +Cerulein	Ethanol diet (0%-36% of total calories) for the total 5weeks and cerulein(20μg/kg b.wt. i.p) thrice a week for last 3weeks to induce CP
V- Group: Ethanol +Cerulein+ HAELR	Ethanol and cerulein + co-administration of 100mg/kg b.wt. of HAELR orally for last 3weeks
VI- Group: Ethanol +Cerulein+ GZ	Ethanol and cerulein + co-administration of10mg/kg b.wt. of GZ orally for last 3weeks

4.10.1 Biochemical Analysis

4.10.1.1 Assay of pancreatic marker enzymes

(a) Assay of Lipase activity (LIP UV:01P)

Lipase activity was determined by the standard protocol provided in the assay kit manual.

$$\text{Triolein} + 2H_2O \xrightarrow{\text{Lipase}} \text{Monoglyceride} + 2\ \text{Oleic acid}$$

Reconstitution of Calibrator

The calibrator provided in the manual was made up with 1 ml of DH2O and left to stay for 10min.

This assay was conducted in serum

Experimental procedure

Two-test tubes were taken and marked, Calibrator “C” and Test “T”.

Order of contents	C	T
Provided-lipase-reagent	1ml	1ml
Reconstituted-calibrator	0.04ml	-
Study-sample	-	0.04ml

Both the tubes were kept at RT for 4min and starting absorbance of C&T were measured at 340nm. Around 5 min later, second absorbance of C&T were measured. Difference in absorbance ΔA for both C&T was found.

For Calibrator $\Delta AC = A_2C - A_1C$

For Test $\Delta AT = A_2T - A_1T$

Lipase = ($\Delta AT/\Delta AC$) X Concentration of calibrator

Where, Concentration of calibrator = 302 U/L [supplied in kit-manual].

Result

Results were expressed as IU/L

(b) Assay of amylase activity (AMY DS:01P)

Amylase activity was determined by the standard protocol provided in the kit manual.

$$\text{CNP-Gal-G2} + H_2O \xrightarrow{\alpha \text{ amylase}} \text{CNP} + \text{Gal-G2}$$

This assay was conducted in serum

Experimental procedure

A test tube was taken and marked "T"

Order of contents	T
Provided-amylase-reagent	1ml
Study-sample	0.02ml

Starting absorbance A0 was measured after 1min, and measurement was done after every 1, 2 and 3min at 405nm. The mean absorbance difference in one minute (ΔA/min) was calculated.

Amylase activity $= \Delta A/min \times 3954$

Result

Results were expressed as IU/L

4.10.1.2 Determination of oxidative stress markers and antioxidants

Levels of cellular oxidative stress were measured through estimations of total peroxide content (TP), total antioxidant capacity (TAC) and oxidative stress index (OSI). Levels of antioxidants like GSH, GPx, SOD, CAT, TBARS and 4-HNE were also estimated.

(a) Determination of TP

Determination of TP →**Miyazawa, 1989**

Assay-principle

Oxidation of ferrous ion to ferric ion by peroxides in study specimens produce ferric-xylenol-orange-complex which was read at 560 nm.

Reagents required

1. FOX2 reagent→ 250mM ammonium ferrous sulfate+ 100mM xylenol orange+ 25mM H2SO4+ 4mM butylated hydroxy toluene were dissolved in 90% methanol.

2. H_2O_2 → 0.06μM in DH2O

This assay was conducted in plasma

Experimental procedure

To 0.2ml of study-sample,1.8ml of prepared FOX2 reagent was added. The contents were left aside for 30min. Centrifugation was carried out at 12,000g for about 10 min. The obtained supernatant was read at 560nm. FOX2 reagent alone served as reference blank.

Result

Results were expressed as μmol/l

(b) Determination of total antioxidant capacity (TAC)

Determination of TAC →**Miller, 1993**.

Assay principle

The loss of colour by ABTS& study-sample mixture was read at 734 nm. The % inhibition was noted as a function of antioxidant concentration. Trolox was the reference standard used.

Reagents required

1. ABTS-stock→7mM

2. $ABTS^+$ dilution-1→ 7mM/I ABTS stock + 2.45mM/l potassium persulfate and incubated, protecting from light, at RT for 12-16h.

3. $ABTS^{\cdot +}$ dilution-2→ ABTS stock solution was diluted with the phosphate buffered saline (5mM, pH 7.4) to an absorbance of 0.70 at 743nm.

4. Standard trolox→ 60nM

This assay was conducted in plasma

Procedure

To 10μl of study-sample, 1ml of $ABTS^{\cdot +}$ dilution-2 was added and its absorbance was measured for 6 minutes at 730nm.

Result

Results were expressed as μmol trolex eq./l

(c) Oxidative stress index (OSI)

It is calculated as represented below, as the ratio of TP& TAC.

OSI = [(Total peroxides, μmol L^{-1}) / (TAC, μmol Trolox equivalent L^{-1}) x 100]

(d) Estimation of glutathione (GSH)

GSH →**Moron, 1979**.

Principle

When DTNB was mixed with compounds having functional-sulfydryl groups, 2-nitro-5-thiobenzoic acid (TNB), an yellow coloured product develops, which can be read at 412nm. It is proportional to the GSH present in the sample.

Reagents required

1. GSH-Standard→ 10mg of GSH in 100ml DH2O.

   Concentration → 100µg/ml

2. Phosphate buffer (0.2M, pH 8)

3. DTNB 0.6mM

4. TCA 5% (ice-cold)

This assay was conducted in serum, tissue homogenate and mitochondrial isolates

Experimental procedure

An aliquot of study-sample and an equal volume of TCA were added to each other and centrifuged at 4000rpm for 10min. To 1ml of supernatant, phosphate buffer(1ml) and DTNB(2ml) were added. Reagent blank was made likewise without study-sample and with TCA instead. The colour developed was read at 412nm against reagent blank in spectrophotometer. Various concentrations of standard GSH: 10 µg to 50µg, were prepared and treated likewise during the estimation.

Result

The amount of GSH in serum was expressed as mg/dL.

The amount of GSH in pancreatic tissue was expressed as mg/g protein.

The amount of GSH in mitochondrial isolate was expressed as mg/g protein.

(e) Estimation of glutathione peroxidase (GPx)

Estimation of glutathione peroxidase GPx →**Flohe & Gunzler, 1984**.

Principle

Enzyme source is initially mixed with hydrogen peroxide and glutathione. The reaction is allowed to proceed and the remaining GSH content is estimated by Ellman's reaction.

Required reagents

1. Phosphate buffer (0.2M pH 8)
2. DTNB→ 0.6mM
3. TrisHCl buffer (0.4M pH 7)
4. Glutathione 2mM
5. H2O2 1mM
6. TCA 10%
7. EDTA 0.4mM
8. Sodium azide solution 10mM

This assay was conducted in serum, tissue homogenate and mitochondrial isolates

Procedure

EDTA (0.2ml), sodium azide (0.1ml), study-sample (0.2ml), and phosphate buffer (0.2ml) were added to each other. To these contents, GSH(0.2ml) and H_2O_2 (0.1ml) were added, mixed thoroughly and kept at RT for 10min. The chemical reaction was then stopped with 0.5ml of TCA and centrifuged at 4000rpm for 10min. To 1ml of supernatant, 1ml of phosphate buffer and 2ml of DTNB reagent were added and mixed. GSH remaining was estimated by Ellman's reaction at 412nm in spectrophotometer.

Result

The activity of GPx in serum was expressed as U/L.

The amount of GPx in pancreatic tissue was expressed as nM GSH oxidized/min/ mg protein.

The amount of GPx in mitochondrial isolate was expressed as nM GSH oxidized/min/ mg

(f) Assay of SOD

Assay of activity of SOD →**Kakkar, 1984**.

Assay-principle

The inhibition of reduction of NBT in the presence of PMS and NADH to blue coloured formazan is measured at 560 nm.

Reagents required

1. Sodium pyrophosphate buffer (0.025M pH 8.3)
2. PMS→186 μM PMS in 100ml of DH2O.
3. NBT→300μM in buffer
4. n-butanol
5. NADH: 780μM in buffer

This assay was conducted in serum, tissue homogenate and mitochondrial isolates

Experimental procedure

Enzyme source(0.4ml), DH2O(1.0ml), sodium pyrophosphate buffer(1.2ml), PMS(0.1ml) and NBT(0.3ml) were mixed with each other. The chemical reaction was initiated by the addition of NADH (0.3ml) and the contents were kept aside at RT for 90 seconds. To halt the reaction, 1ml glacial acetic acid was used. 4ml of n-butanol was added to all the tubes, allowed to stand for 10min, centrifuged and butanol layer was carefully separated. The colour intensity was measured at 560nm in spectrophotometer. Control tube had all the mentioned contents except the enzyme source. Concentration of enzyme that gives 50% inhibition of chromogen formation per minute was considered as one unit.

Result

The activity of enzyme in serum was expressed as U/L.

The activity of enzyme in pancreatic tissue was expressed as units / mg protein.

The activity of enzyme in mitochondrial isolate was expressed as units / mg protein.

(g) Assay of Catalase

Assay of catalase activity →**Aebi,1984**.

Assay-principle

The enzyme catalase present in the study-samples decomposes H_2O_2 to H_2O and O_2 for different time periods. The chemical reaction is stopped at specific time intervals with dichromate& acetic acid solution and the remaining H_2O_2 is determined. Dichromate in acetic acid gets reduced to chromic acetate if heated along with hydrogen peroxide with the formation of perchloric acid as an unstable intermediate. Thus formed chromic acetate is measured at 610nm in a colorimeter.

Reagents required

1. Phosphate buffer (0.01M pH 7)
2. H2O2→ 0.2M
3. Stock dichromate: acetic acid reagent→ 5% K2Cr2O7 and CH_3 COOH (1:3)
4. Working dichromate: acetic acid solution→ The stock was diluted five number of times using DH2O to obtain working dichromate/acetic acid solution.

This assay was conducted in serum, tissue homogenate and mitochondrial isolates

Experimental procedure

H_2O_2 (0.5ml), buffer(1ml), DH2O(0.4ml), study-sample (0.2 ml) and dichromate/acetic acid reagent(2ml) were added to each other. Aliquots were drawn after 0,30,60,90 seconds of incubation. In case of control tube, the study-sample was added only after the addition of acid reagent. All the test tubes were heated for 10min and the colour developed was measured at 610nm.

Result

The activity of catalase in serum was expressed as U/L.

The activity of catalase in pancreatic tissue was expressed as µM of H2O2 decomposed/min/mg protein.

The activity of catalase in mitochondrial isolate was expressed as µM of H2O2 decomposed/min/mg protein.

(h) Estimation of TBARS

Estimation of TBARS→ **Draper and Hadley,1990**.

Assay-principle

MDA, a lipid peroxidation product reacts with TBA to produce a coloured product, whose intensity at 533nm, is proportional to the levels of lipid peroxidation products in study-samples.

Reagents required

1. Stock MDA→80μl of 1, 1', 3, 3'-tetramethoxy propane / malonaldehyde bis(dimethyl acetal) in 100ml DH2O.

   Concentration = 5μM/ml

2. Working MDA→1ml stock diluted to 100ml with DH2O.

   Concentration = 50nM/ml

3. TBA→0.67% of TBA was prepared with 50% glacial acetic acid.

4. n-butanol

5. $H_3PW_{12}O_{40}$→10%

6. H_2SO_4 →4M

This assay was conducted in tissue homogenate and mitochondrial isolates

Experimental procedure

Aliquots of study-samples, 4M H_2SO_4(0.5ml), 10% PTA(0.4ml) and DH2O(1ml) were added to each, incubated at RT for 5 min and centrifuged at 3000rpm for 10min. The obtained pellet was mixed with 1ml of 4M H_2SO_4& 0.15ml of 10% PTA and then incubated for 5 min at RT. Test-tubes were centrifuged again at 3000rpm for 10min. The obtained pellet was suspended again in 2ml of DH2O. 0.5ml of TBA was then added, mixed thoroughly and the contents were kept in boiling water bath for an hour. The test-tubes were cooled and 2.5ml of butanol was added (if turbidity observed) and mixed thoroughly for a minute. The test-tubes were centrifuged and the absorbance of obtained supernatant was read at 533nm.

Result

The values were expressed as nM/mg protein in pancreatic tissue homogenate.

The values were expressed as nM/mg protein in mitochondrial isolates.

(i) Estimation of 4-hydroxynonenol (4-HNE)

Estimation of 4-HNE →**Kinter,1994.**

Reagents required

1. Stock standard→1mg of 6.4 μM 4HNE was taken in 6.4ml of methanol to produce 1mM solution.

$$[4HNE] = (A_{220}/13750) \times 50$$

Where, A_{220} is the absorbance at 220nm relative to a methanol blank,

13750 is the molar extinction coefficient for 4HNE in methanol and

50 is the dilution factor.

2. Working standard→ Suitable dilutions were made with stock standard to achieve a concentration of 0.1mM
3. HCl →0.5M
4. Dinitrophenyl hydrazine→100mg in 100ml of 0.5M hydrochloric acid
5. TCA 10%
6. Hexane
7. Methanol

This assay was conducted in tissue homogenate and mitochondrial isolates

Experimental procedure

To 2ml of study-sample, 10% TCA(1.5ml) was added and centrifugation was carried out at 3000 rpm for 30min. To 2 ml of obtained-filterate, 1ml of DNPH was added and kept at RT for 60min. Extraction of contents was done using hexane and the extract was kept for evaporation at 40°C. Methanol(2ml) was then added to the extract and was read at 350nm. Methanol alone served as blank.

Result

The concentration of 4-HNE was expressed as μM/g protein.

4.10.1.3 Assessment of inflammatory markers

Levels of myeloperoxidase (MPO), caspase-1, IL-1β, IL-18, and NF-kB were determined to evaluate the progression of inflammation.

(a) Determination of myeloperoxidase activity

Determination of myeloperoxidase activity →**Bradley, 1982**.

Reagents required

1. Phosphate buffer (10mM pH 6)
2. Potassium phosphate buffer (50mM pH 6)
3. Cetrimonium bromide →0.5%
4. H_2O_2 →0.0005%
5. 0-dianisidine dihydrochloride →0.167g/l

This assay was conducted in tissue homogenate

Experimental procedure

A small portion of pancreas was weighed and homogenized in 50mM phosphate buffer (pH 6), with 0.5% bromide. The study-samples were centrifuged at

17,000 X g for 15min (4°C). Aliquots of obtained-supernatant were mixed with 0.167 mg/mL of o-dianisidine &0.0005% H_2O_2 solution. 10mM phosphate buffer (pH 6) was used to prepare this solution. The contents were read at 460nm in spectrophotometer and change in absorbance was noted for about 4 min at 30second intervals. One unit of MPO activity was considered as that which degrades 1mmol of peroxide per min at 25°C.

Result

MPO activity was expressed as U/mg protein.

(b) Assay of caspase-1(Assay kit: ab39470)

Assay-principle

The breakage of the peptide by caspase produces the chromphore pNA, that can be quantitated at 405nm. The caspase activity in the cell lysate is directly proportional to the colour.

This assay was conducted in serum

Experimental procedure

The pancreatic tissue homogenate was centrifuged at 250 x g for 10 min. To the obtained pellet, lysis buffer was added and incubated on ice for 10min.The contents were centrifuged at 10,000 g for 1 min. The obtained-supernatant (protein concentration: 2-4 mg/ml) was collected and kept on ice. To a 96 well microplate, 50μl of supernatant,10μl of DTT,50μl of 2X reaction buffer and 5μl of YVAD-pNA were added sequentially to each well. The microplates were incubated at RT for 2 hours and read at 405nm in a microplate reader.

Results

The level of caspase-1 in serum was expressed as pg/ml.

(c) Assay of interleukin-1β (IL-1β, Assay kit: ab100767)

Assay-principle

Quantitative sandwich enzyme immunoassay technique: A monoclonal antibody specific for interleukin-1β was pre-coated onto a microplate. Standards and samples are pipetted into the wells and any interleukin-1β present gets bound by the immobilized antibody. The colour developed is proportional to the amount of interleukin-1β bound, which is measured.

This assay was conducted in serum

Wash buffer

20ml of wash buffer concentrate was diluted with DH2O to prepare 500ml of wash buffer.

Substrate solution

Colour reagents A & B were mixed with each other in equal volumes and kept away from light. 200μl of the resultant mixture was used per well.

IL-1β standard

IL-1β standard was reconstituted with calibrator **(Figure 4.1)** to produce a stock solution of 250 pg/ml. The standards were kept aside for 15 min. 500 μl of calibrator diluent was pipetted into each tube. The stock solution was used for dilution series. The undiluted IL-1β standard (250 pg/ml) was considered the high standard. The appropriate calibrator diluent was considered the zero standard (0 pg/ml).

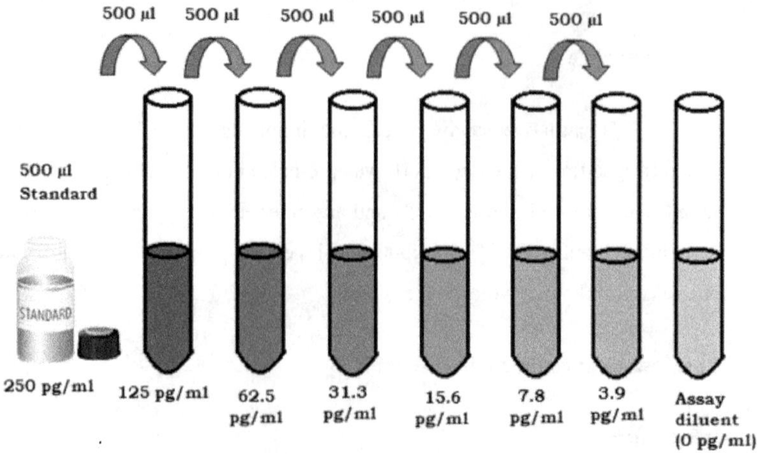

Figure 4.1 Serial dilutions of IL-1β standards

Experimental procedure

50µl of assay diluent ,200µl of standard or study-sample were added to each well. The wells were then covered with an adhesive strip and incubated for 2 hours at RT. Each well was washed thrice with 400 µl wash buffer. Finally, the micro-plates were blotted against clean paper towels to remove wash buffer. 200µl of IL-1β conjugate was added to each well, covered using adhesive strip and incubated for 2 hours at RT. Similar wash steps were performed again. 200µl of substrate was then added to each well, incubated at RT for 20min, away from light. 50µl of stop solution was added and the colour change from blue to yellow was recorded. The OD of each well was determined within 30 minutes at 450nm in a microplate reader.

Results

The level of IL-1β was expressed in pg/ml

(d) Assay of interleukin-18 (IL-18, Assay kit: KRC2341)

Assay-principle

Solid phase sandwich ELISA technique: A polyclonal antibody specific for Rat IL-18 was pre-coated onto a microplate. Standards of IL-18, control and study-samples were pipetted into wells. Streptavidin-Peroxidase is the enzyme provided, which binds to the biotinylated antibody to complete the four-member sandwich. After the second incubation followed by washing to remove the entire unbound enzyme, a substrate solution is added, which is acted upon by the bound enzyme to give colour. The intensity of this coloured product is directly proportional to the concentration of rat IL-18 present in the study-sample.

This assay was conducted in serum

Wash solution

One volume of the wash buffer concentrate (25X) was diluted with 24 volumes of deionized water to make working wash buffer.

Conjugate solution

10 μl of Streptavidin-HRP concentrate (100X) was diluted with 1 ml of Streptavidin-HRP diluent to prepare Streptavidin-HRP working solution.

IL-18 Standards

The Rat IL-18 standard was calibrated against a recombinant baculovirus protein.

- Standard was reconstituted to 5,000 pg/ml with standard diluent buffer.
- 0.1 ml of the reconstituted standard was added to a tube containing 0.4 ml standard diluent buffer and marked as 1,000 pg/ml and mixed.
- 0.25 ml of standard diluent buffer was added to each of six tubes labeled as 500, 250, 125, 62.5, 31.3 and 15.6 pg/ml of rat IL-18.
- Serial dilutions of the standard were carried out **(Figure 4.2)**

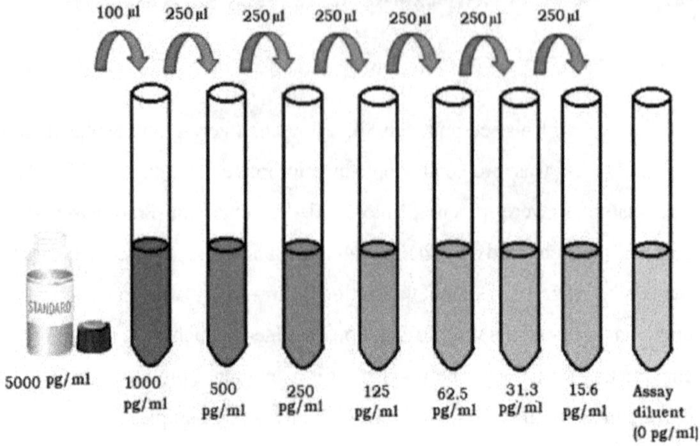

Figure 4.2 Serial dilutions of IL-18 standards

Assay procedure

Sample incubation

A volume of 100 µl of standard diluent buffer was added to the zero standard well. Wells for chromogen blank were left empty. 100 µl of standards, study-samples and control were added to the appropriate wells. 50 µl of incubation buffer was added to the zero standard well and to the wells containing standards and serum, incubated for 2 hours at RT.

Washing

The wells were washed thrice by completely aspirating the existing solution from the wells.

Conjugate incubation

A volume of 100 µl biotinylated rat IL-18 biotin conjugate solution was added into each well, leaving out the chromogen blank and incubated for 1 hour at RT.

Washing

The wells were washed four times by completely decanting the solution from the wells.

Substrate incubation

A volume of 100 µl Streptavidin-HRP working solution was added to each well, leaving out the chromogen blank. The plates were covered using plate cover and incubated for 30 minutes at RT. The wells were washed thrice like mentioned before. 100 µl of stabilized chromogen was added to each well and the liquid in the wells turned blue. The contents were incubated in dark at RT for 30 min.

Stop reaction

A volume of 100 µl stop solution was added to each well. The colour of the solution in the well changes from blue to yellow. The absorbance was read in each well after adding the stop solution within 2 hours at 450 nm against a chromogen blank.

Results

The level of IL-18 was expressed in pg/ml

(e) Determination of NF-κB

The mRNA expression levels of NF-κB were measured in pancreas by qRT-PCR analysis in molecular studies.

4.10.1.4 Assessment of ER stress markers

The mRNA expression levels of UPR components like ATF4, GRP78, CHOP and XBP1 were measured in pancreas by qRT-PCR analysis in molecular studies.

MOLECULAR STUDIES

Quantitative real time polymerase chain reaction (qRT-PCR)

RT-PCR analysis was performed to determine the mRNA expression of ER stress markers ATF4, GRP78, CHOP, XBP1 and inflammatory marker NF-κB levels in pancreatic tissue. β-actin was used as the house keeping gene.

After animal sacrifice, 50mg of the pancreas was excised from the rat and suspended immediately into the RNA later solution. Using RNeasy Miniprep kit (No. 74104), the total RNA was extracted from the study-sample.

Study-principle

The RNeasy technology incorporates selective binding properties of a silica-based membrane with microspin technology. Up to 100 μg of RNA longer than 200 bases that binds to the RNeasy silica membrane in the presence of a specialized high-salt buffer system was used. Study-samples are initially lysed and then homogenized with guanidine-thiocyanate–containing buffer, which inactivates RNases to protect intact RNA. Binding is enhanced with ethanol and the study-sample is applied to RNeasy Mini spin column. RNA binds to the membrane, while washing off any contaminants. RNA is then eluted in 30–100 μl water. In this efficient procedure, RNAs < 200 nucleotides are selectively excluded.

Experimental procedure

Approximately, 30 mg of pancreas was weighed and added to 600 μL Buffer RLT. The tissue was then homogenized to obtain uniform homogeneity. The obtained-lysate was centrifuged for 3 min at 12,000 rpm. The supernatant was collected. 700 μL of the obtained-lysate was applied to an RNeasy spin column placed in a 2 ml collection tube and centrifuged for 15 s at ≥8000 x *g* (≥10,000 rpm).

A volume of 700 μl Buffer RW1 was added to the RNeasy spin column and centrifugation performed for 15 s at ≥8000 x *g* (≥10,000 rpm) in order to wash the column membrane. The washing procedure is repeated two times discarding the flow-through, in between. Finally, the RNeasy spin column was kept in 1.5 ml collection tube and 30–50 µl RNase-free water was directly added to the spin column membrane and centrifuged for 1 min at ≥ 8000 x *g* (≥10,000 rpm) to elute the RNA.

Determination of RNA purity and concentration

RNA was quantified using a spectrophotometer and the purity of the sample was determined using A260/280 ratio.

Synthesis of cDNA

Required volumes of components of the RT-mastermix were mixed, at the cold environment. The prepared master mix was distributed into 0.2ml vials. To each vial, 200ng/10 µL of the RNA sample was added, making up the final volume to 20µL, using nuclease-free water. The samples were then loaded into the thermal cycler, setting up the volume to 20µL. The program was performed and resultant cDNA was stored at -20°C.

RT master mix (per 20-µL reaction)

Contents	Volume
10X Reaction Buffer	2µL
Primer Mix	2µL
100mM dNTP's	0.8µL
Reverse Trasncriptase	1µL
RNA	200ng/10µL
Nuclease-free water	4.2µL
Total per reaction	20µL

PCR program for cDNA synthesis

	STEP 1	STEP 2	STEP 3	STEP 4
Temperature(°C)	25	37	85	4
Time	10 min	120 min	5 min	∞

qRT-PCR :

qRT-PCR was performed using SYBR Green. The expression of the following genes in the samples were assessed:

- ***Actb*** (β-actin) – as reference gene
- ***ATF4*** (ATF4)
- ***GRP78*** (GRP78)
- ***CHOP*** (CHOP)
- ***XbpI*** (XBP1)
- ***Nfkb1*** (NF-κB)

Experimental procedure:

The 2X premix provided was thoroughly mixed. The reaction master mix with each primer set was made ready for required number of samples. All the preparations were done on ice. All reactions were performed in duplicate or triplicate along with control. All the sample tubes were covered with the provided optical film (Agilent: #401425). Sample tubes were initially centrifuged, ensuring contents to settle down and also to eliminate air bubbles. The samples were loaded onto the RT-PCR machine (Stratagene Mx3000P) and the appropriate program was run. The resultant qPCR products were stored at -20°C.

qPCR product analysis by agarose gel electrophoresis

The RT-PCR products obtained from the previous step were now loaded on a 1.5% agarose gel to check amplification specificity. 10μL of the amplified product was mixed with 1μL of 10X loading dye and loaded into the wells along with 1μL of molecular weight marker (100-1000bp ladder). The electrophoresis was carried out at 100V in 0.5X TBE buffer. UV illuminator was used to analyze the gel and the products obtained were compared with the ladder. The qPCR data was collected and analyzed on MxPro qPCR software for Cq values.

Oligonucleotide primers used for qPCR

Gene	Forward primer	Reverse primer
β-actin	5′-CACCAACTGGGACGACAT-3’	5′-ACAGCCTGGATAGCAACG-3’
ATF4	5′-TGAAAGAGAAGGCAGATT-3’	5′-TGAAAGAGAAGGCAGATT-3’
CHOP	5′-TGTTCTCTATTCGTTCCTAA-3’	5′-CCACCATCCTGAACTATT-3’
GRP78	5′-AATCAAGGTCTACGAAGG-3’	5′-AACACTGGTCCAACTAAG-3’
XBP1	5′-AACCTCTTAGATGACTTCCA-3’	5′-AGGCTGAACGATAACTGT-3’
NF-kB	5′-CAATCTTGATGTCATTCG-3’	5′-AAGTGTAATCCAATAGCA-3’

SYBR green PCR master mixture

Components	Volume (µl)
SYBR Green mix (2x)	10 µl
Forward primer	1 µl
Reverse primer	1 µl
Template (cDNA)	1 µl
50X Rox- Reference Dye	0.4 µl
Sterile water	6.6 µl
Total volume	20 µl

Program for SYBR-based qPCR

Stages	Temperature	Time
Initial Denaturation	95°C	10 min
Denaturation	95°C	30 sec
Annealing	60°C	60 sec
Repetition cycles	40 cycles	

4.10.1.5 Functional aspects of mitochondria

(a) Isolation of Mitochondria

Principle

The mitochondria from pancreatic tissue samples from different experimental groups, have been isolated using this isolation kit employing differential centrifugation as the basic principle. Initially, washed and homogenized pancreatic tissue was suspended in the isolation buffer provided and centrifugation was carried out at low speed to remove any cell debris and bulky large organelles (in, spin-1). Spin-1 was carried at 1000g for 10min at 4°C.The obtained- supernatant was centrifuged at 12,000g for 15min at 4°C (spin-2). The pellet was washed by re-suspending in the isolation buffer and protease inhibitor. Then centrifugation was again carried out at 12,000g for 15min, collected the pellet and the process was repeated by re-suspending the pellet in the isolation buffer and protease inhibitor to finally collect the isolated, intact and active mitochondria (in, spin-2).

Reagents included in the kit

Content	Quantity
Wash buffer	30ml
Isolation buffer	100ml

Wash buffer and Isolation buffer should always be stored at 4°C.

Reagents and equipment needed

1. Double DH2O
2. Protease inhibitor cocktail (PI) (ab201111)
3. Standard protein assay
4. Homogenizer (2 mL size) with pestles
5. High speed benchtop centrifuge

6. 2.0 mL micro tubes
7. Weighing balance and other standard lab equipments

Experimental procedure

The overall procedure is to rupture the cells of the pancreatic tissue, centrifuge to remove large organelles, and then centrifuge to isolate the mitochondria. Weighed around 0.5g of the pancreatic tissue and washed the tissue samples two times with 1.5ml of the chilled wash buffer provided. Minced the tissue into small pieces and ruptured using chilled homogenizer, by adding up to 2ml of the chilled isolation buffer. Care has to be taken without overdoing on ice.

During spin-1, the tissue homogenate was shifted to one or more 2ml centrifuge tubes as needed. By filling each centrifuge tube with 2ml of isolation buffer, the homogenate was centrifuged at 1000g for 10min at 4°C. The supernatant obtained was saved and the pellet was discarded.

During spin-2, the supernatant from the previous spin was shifted to new centrifuge tubes, added the isolation buffer and centrifuged again at 12,000g for 15min at 4°C to collect the pellet. The pellet was washed, re-suspended in 1ml isolation buffer with 10 μL protease inhibitor. Then centrifuged again at 12,000g for 15min at 4°C to collect the pellet. Pellets were washed and re-suspended in 500 μL of isolation buffer with protease inhibitor. The resultant aliquots of mitochondrial suspension were freezed at -80°C until use. Concentration of protein in isolated mitochondria was then quantified using Bradford assay.

Result

Isolates of mitochondria from various pancreatic tissue extracts were obtained.

(b) Determination of mitochondrial oxidative stress

Oxidative stress level in various mitochondrial isolates was assessed through estimation of GSH (Moron,1979); GPx (Flohé and Günzler,1984); SOD

(Kakkar, 1984); CAT (Aebi, 1984); MDA/TBARS (Draper and Hadley, 1990) and 4-HNE (Kinter, 1984). The methods were described in earlier sections.

(c) Determination of mitochondrial calcium $[Ca^{2+}]_m$

The concentration of calcium in the mitochondrial isolates of various experimental groups was determined by using fura-2 AM, a ratiometric calcium indicator.

Principle

The ratio of the emitted intensities by fura-2 AM at 340- and 380-nm excitations is used to determine the concentration of Ca^{2+}.

Reagents required

1. Sucrose solution 0.25 M
2. EGTA 1 mM
3. Tris buffer 20 mM, pH 7.4
4. Hanks' balanced salt solution (HBSS with Ca^{2+}): 137 mM of NaCl, 5.37 mM of KCl, 0.81 mM of $MgSO_4$, 0.44 mM of KH_2PO_4, 0.37 mM of Na_2HPO_4, 1.37 mM of $CaCl_2$, 5.56 mM of glucose (pH was adjusted to 7.2 with 10 mM 4-(2-hydroxyethyl)-1-piperazineethane sulfonic acid).
5. Fura-2 AM: 1 mg of fura-2 AM was dissolved in 1 ml dimethyl sulfoxide to prepare a stock solution of fura-2 AM. For the experiment, an aliquot of stock solution was diluted to 10 μM in modified Hanks' balanced salt solution (HBSS with Ca^{2+}) just before loading.

Equipment

ELICO's SL-174 spectrofluorometer for the measurement.

This assay was conducted in mitochondrial isolates

Experimental procedure

Mitochondrial isolates were initially suspended in 0.25 M sucrose solution, that contains 1 mM EGTA and 20 mM Tris (pH 7.4). Then they were loaded with 10 μM fura-2 AM in the buffer, incubated for 10 minutes at RT. The isolates were washed twice and resuspended in the same HBSS buffer. Calcium concentration in the mitochondrial isolates was measured at 37°C by monitoring fura-2 AM fluorescence in spectrofluorimeter with the excitation at 340nm and 380nm and emission at 510nm [Hotta Y,2001] [Trenker M,2008].

Result

The calcium concentrations were calculated and expressed in nM by conversion of the obtained values into ratio, according to the below mentioned formula [Grynkiewicz G,1985].

$$\left[Ca^{2+}\right]=K_d\left(\frac{R-R_{\min}}{R_{\max}-R}\right)\left(\frac{S_{f2}}{S_{b2}}\right)$$

(d) Determination of Complex-1

Principle

Complex-1 (NADH dehydrogenase or E.C.1.6.5.3) activity in mitochondria was determined using an assay kit, which relies on colorimetry principle. The kit basically recognizes NADH dependent activity of complex-1, in cell or tissue extracts or isolates. Specific antibodies for the complex-1 were precoated in the provided microplate of the kit. When the samples are added to the microplate, and the target has been immobilized inside the well, oxidation of NADH to NAD^+ occurs, followed by the simultaneous reduction of provided dye. The functional status of complex-1 is thus elicited based on the activity shown.

Reagents included in the kit

Item	Quantity	Pre-preparatory storage	Post-preparatory storage
20X Wash Buffer	25 mL	4°C	4°C
10X Blocking Buffer	10 mL	4°C	4°C
10X Detergent	1 mL	4°C	4°C
20X NADH (40 mM after addition of H2O)	1 vial	4°C	-80°C
100XDye(lyophilized)	1 vial	4°C	-80°C
96-well microplate (12 x 8 well strips)	1	4°C	4°C

Reagents and equipment needed

1. Microplate reader, which can read OD 450nm
2. Double DH2O
3. Suitable laboratory glassware and pipettes for reagent and buffer preparation

Reagent preparation

20X Wash Buffer: Prepared 1X Buffer by diluting 20X Buffer in double DH2O. 500 mL of 1X Buffer was made by combining 25 mL of 20X Buffer and 475 mL of double DH2O. The contents were mixed thoroughly. The prepared buffer is stored at 4°C and equilibrated to RT just before using.

10X Blocking Solution: Diluted 10X Blocking Solution in Buffer to prepare Incubation Solution. 100 mL of Incubation solution was made by combining 10 mL of 10X Blocking Solution with 90 mL of Buffer. The combined contents were mixed thoroughly and gently. The prepared Incubation buffer is stored at 4°C and equilibrated to RT before use.

10X Detergent: It is a ready to use detergent stored at 4°C. But equilibration to RT is needed before using.

20X NADH: Reconstituted the lyophilized NADH in 1.1 mL of double DH2O and mixed thoroughly until dissolved, 40 mM solution was made. Stored at -80°C and always to be kept on ice while using

100X Dye: Reconstituted the dye in 250 μL of double DH2O and mix thoroughly until dissolved. Stored at -80°C. Kept on ice while in use.

Assay solution: Prepared 1.75 mL per strip of Assay Solution according to the kit manual and used for the assay.

96-well microplate (12 x 8-well strips): It is a ready to use microplate. This plate can be broken as needed, into 12 separate 8-well strips. Stored at 4°C and equilibrated to RT before use.

This assay was conducted in mitochondrial isolates

Experimental procedure

Around 200 μL of mitochondrial isolates from various pancreatic tissue samples, were loaded onto the microplate provided. 200 μL of 1X Incubation buffer was added to buffer only wells, which stands as control. Contents were then incubated for 3hours at RT. Turned the plate over, to empty the contents and shaked to let out any remaining liquid. Blotted the plate down on a tissue towel. The wells were then washed with 300 μL of 1X Buffer solution. 200 μL of assay solution was then added to each well avoiding bubble formation and OD was measured at 450nm. The measurement was done in the microplate reader in a kinetic mode for 30minutes with a time interval of 1min, at RT.

Result

The activity is expressed as, the change in absorbance per minute per amount of sample loaded into the well.

4.10.1.6 Histopathological studies

Histopathology is the study that involves examination of tissues or cells under a microscope.

Experimental procedure

Tissue resection and fixation: A small portion of the test organs were placed in the fixative (10% formal-saline) overnight.

Dehydration: After fixation, the tissue was dehydrated using isopropyl alcohol (IPA).

IPA concentration	Time-period
70% IPA	1 hour
70% IPA	1 hour
85% IPA	1 hour
95% IPA	1 hour
100% IPA	1 hour
100% IPA	1 hour

Infiltration: 100% IPA was removed and the vial was filled using melted paraffin and equilibration was carried out for an hour at 58°C.

Embedding: The paraffin from previous step was emptied and the corresponding tissue blocks were transferred to the mold and was filled again with paraffin. Solidification of the paraffin takes place when kept RT and was used further.

Sectioning: Sectioning was done using microtome, which is a specialized precision cutting instrument, that accurately slices the embedded tissues. The excess paraffin in the tissue block was removed initially and tissue sections of around 5-10μm thick were cut with microtome. Thus obtained tissue sections were then prepared for mounting onto microscopic slides.

Mounting: The tissue sections were now kept in a pre-warmedsolution of adhesive, Sta-On. It is a liquid and non-coagulating adhesive. A clean and dry microscope slide was slightly immersed into the Sta-On solution and taken back out. This causes adherence of tissue sections to microscopic slides which were now dried overnight.

Clearing and staining: Clearing-step was conducted with the solvent Clearene, that dissolves the paraffin and enables permanent adherence of tissue sections to the microscopic slides.

Step-1	:	3 min
Step-2	:	2 min
Step-3	:	1 min
100% IPA	:	30 sec
85% IPA	:	30 sec
70% IPA	:	30 sec
Tap water	:	30 sec

Two histological stains were used for staining procedure viz. hematoxylin and eosin. Hematoxylin stains the nuclei of the cell, a purple blue colour. Eosin, stains extra-cellular matrix and cytoplasm,a pink colour.

Hematoxylin	:	2 min
Tap water	:	30 sec
Scott's solution (240mM $NaHCO_3$, 1.7mM $MgSO_4$)	:	1 min
Tap water	:	30 sec
Buffer	:	1 min
Tap water	:	30 sec
70% IPA	:	1 min
95% IPA	:	1 min
Eosin Y	:	1 min

Permanent mounting: Lastly, the tissue sections were sealed under a coverslip using resin warmed up a little and kept at RT for 1-2days.

Photomicrography: The normal tissue architecture and histological changes if any, in the hematoxylin and eosin stained tissue sections were photographed at 400X magnification.

4.10.1.7 *Insilico* molecular docking analysis

Target protein identification

Structures of GRP78 and ATF4 were retrieved from UniProt (http://www. uniprot.org/). The crystal structures of GRP78 and ATF4 were downloaded from PDB database and their PDB ids were 5E84 chain A and 1CI6 – A -chain, respectively **(Figure 4.3)**. Further, the structures were visualized using Biovia Discovery studio visualizer (http://accelrys.com/products/discovery-studio/visualization.html).

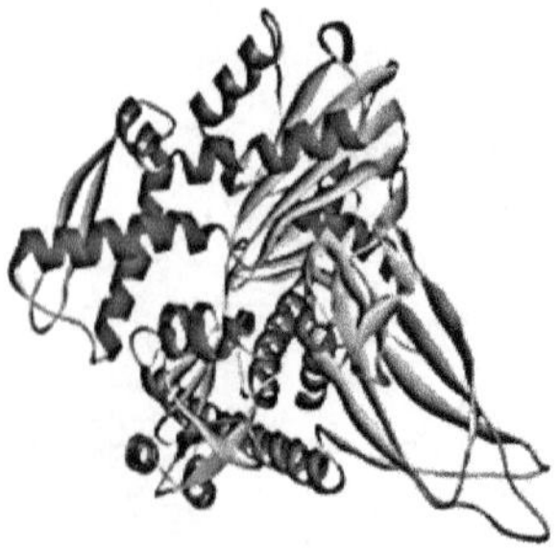

Structure of GRP78

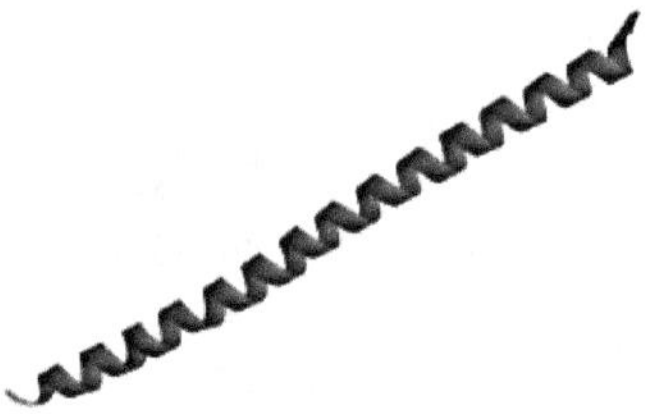

Structure of ATF4-C/EBP BETA BZIP domain

Figure 4.3 Structures of GRP78 and ATF4

Ligand structure preparation

The 2D structure of glycyrrhizin was drawn using ACD chemsketch http://www.acdlabs.com/resources/freeware/chemsketch/) and saved in 3D MDL MOL Format and converted to PDB (http://www.rcsb.org/pdb/home/home.do) format using Open Babel Molecular Converter (http://openbabel.org/ docs/current/ Introduction/

goals.html). The 3D structure of glycyrrhizin (PubChemCID: 14982) was retrieved from PubChem (http://pubchem.ncbi.nlm.nih.gov/) database **(Figure 4.4)**.

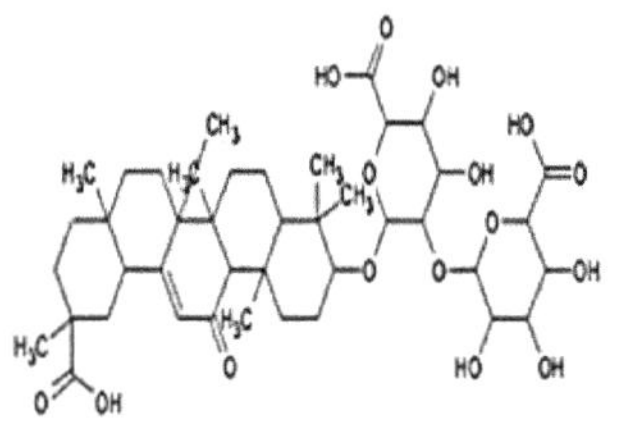

2D Structure of Glycyrrhizin

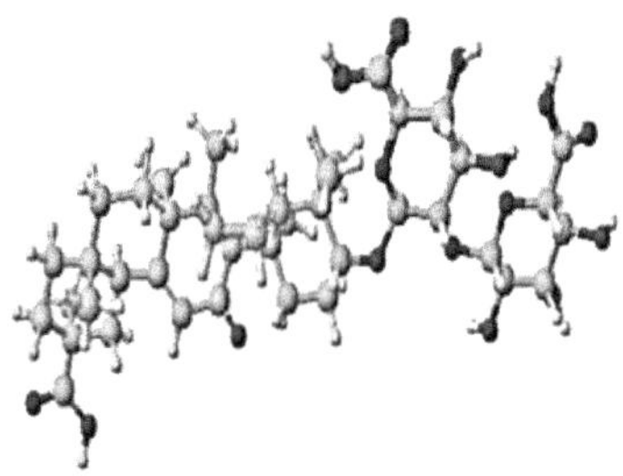

3D Structure of Glycyrrhizin

Figure 4.4 2D and 3D structures of GZ

Molecular Descriptor calculation

Molinspiration online database (http://www.molinspiration.com/) was used to calculate the descriptors of glycrrihizin, such as log P, polar surface area (PSA), molecular weight, number of atoms, number of O or N, number of OH or NH, number of rotatable bonds, volume, drug likeness includes G protein coupled receptors (GPCR) ligand, ion channel modulator, kinase inhibitor and nuclear receptor ligand, and number of violations to Lipinski's rule of Five.

Lipinski's rule of Five

Lipinski's rule of five (**Lipinski, 2004**) defines drug-ability properties of the lead compounds particularly absorption and permeation. The general guidelines are as follows:

LogP <= 5,

molecular weight <= 500 g/mol,

Hydrogen bond donors (sum of NH and OH) <= 5,

number of rotatable bonds (rotb) <= 15

Hydrogen bond acceptors (sum of N and O) <= 10

Compounds violating more than one of the above mentioned guidelines, are more likely to be poorly absorbed.

Tool-Auto dock

The binding energy was calculated using Auto Dock (http://autodock. scripps.edu/resources/tools).

Molecular interaction studies

The molecular interactions were visualized using Acceryls Discovery Studio Visualizer. Default ligand–receptor interaction tool was used to determine hydrogen and hydrophobic interactions. This application runs on Windows and Linux.

4.10.1.8 Statistical analysis

Data were analysed by SPSS software package for Windows v.10. Statistical significance was determined by one-way ANOVA followed by post hoc Bonferroni test and if observed p value is less than 0.05, a statistical significance was recorded. Spearman's rank one-tailed correlation analysis was conducted so as to verify the correlation between the related data sets like GRP78 vs 4-HNE; CHOP vs IL-1 β, [Ca 2+]m and NF-κB; [Ca 2+]m vs TBARS,GSH and complex-1.The correlation coefficient (rs) and its statistical significance level based on exact critical probability (p) values were calculated.

5. RESULTS AND DISCUSSION

CP leads to morphological and functional changes in the pancreas due to the destruction of healthy pancreatic tissue and gradual development of fibrous scar tissue. This functional loss can lead to diabetes mellitus and exocrine pancreatic insufficiency [Zhao X,2020]. Chronic and progressive fibro-inflammation can also lead to many other complications like abscess, upper digestive bleeding, chronic abdominal pain syndrome, metabolic bone disease etc [Ramsey ML,2017]. CP is associated with high morbidity and mortality, and is a major risk factor for various pancreatic cancers and many extra pancreatic malignancies like upper respiratory and digestive tract cancers [Korpela T,2020].

The highly probable and common risk factor for CP is alcohol. Abdominal pain is the most reported symptom of CP and is the main reason to treat the patient immediately [Duggan SN,2016]. Pain can radiate directly to the back, or laterally to the left or right and it can range from several hours to several days. Generally, anti-inflammatory drugs like glucocorticoids and NSAIDs are suggested to minimize and reduce the pain which results from inflammatory processes, during CP. Historically, NSAIDs such as acetylsalicylic acid, diclofenac, indomethacin, ibuprofen, celecoxib, metamizole and piroxicam have been used clinically for the treatment of pancreatic inflammation due to their suppressive effect on COX activity [Wu D,2020].These available treatment regimens were seen to provide, effective but temporary pain relief. They are good in managing complications but are highly ineffective to halt or slow down the advancement of inflammation in pancreas [Conwell DL,2014].

Many similar chronic diseases like cancer, diabetes, cardiovascular, autoimmune, and neurodegenerative disorders, are also closely related with tissue injury and pathological changes, induced by persistent inflammation. The therapeutic approaches for all these chronic conditions, mostly leave more debilitating side effects than the disease itself, summoning the hunt for safer, less toxic, and cost-effective therapeutic alternatives. Exploring the potential of natural products in order to treat inflammatory diseases, paved a way to integrate traditional medicine into modern chronic disease treatment plan [Kim JH,2018]. Herbal drugs were included and constituted in all the officially recognized systems of medicines in India -Ayurveda, Yoga, Unani, Siddha, Homeopathy and Naturopathy. Approximately, 70% of India's 1.1 billion population still use herbal medicine, either alone or in combination with others to improve the efficacy safely [Vaidya AD,2007]. Sen etal., reviewed and enlisted a number of herbal drugs used in Indian traditional medicine since ancient times, highlighting India as a unique place of new drug discovery [Sen S,2017].

In our study, the therapeutic potentials of hydroalcoholic extract of licorice root (HAELR) and its major component glycyrrhizin (GZ), were evaluated against ethanol and cerulein induced CP in rats. CP was induced in rats by repeated Cer injections combined with a sensitizing agent, EtOH. Hyperstimulation with Cer induces pancreatic injury in rats and EtOH administration aggravates this pathological effect towards CP, with clinical presentations like persistent inflammation [Deng,2005]. Various other pathological changes of CP like oxidative stress, ER stress and mitochondrial oxidative stress were also focused.

5.1 Qualitative and Quantitative phytochemical analysis of HAELR

Phytochemical screening was done to detect the presence of wide groups of naturally occurring phytochemicals in HAELR. It was thought that, eliciting the bioactive profile of HAELR is very important before proceeding towards its therapeutic potential.

5.1.1 GCMS analysis of hydroalcoholic extract of licorice root

GCMS is an analytical technique which quantitatively determines phytochemicals in plant extracts, even at very low concentrations. It assists in knowing the significance of traditional herbs and proceeding towards their scientific validation [Al-Rubaye AF,2017]. Using this technique, three compounds were detected in HAELR: 3-hydroxy-3',4',5,7-tetramethoxyflavone, jaceidin triacetate and undecane **(Table 5.1)**.

The GC-MS chromatogram of HAELR was shown in **figure 5.1**. Observation of results indicated the presence of rare flavonoids such as 3-hydroxy-3',4',5,7-tetramethoxyflavone which is documented to be an excellent preventor of lipid peroxidation. The 3-OH group and other electron presenting substituents like OH/- OCH3 groups at positions 5 and 7 are reported to be responsible for its antioxidant activity [Li YL,2017]. The other rare flavonoid [Dhananjayan K,2015] found was jaceidin triacetate which is reported to have modest antioxidative activity by previous studies [Aljancić I,2010]. These compounds might contribute to the antioxidant nature of licorice roots and could have attenuated pathological oxidative stress in pancreas.

Table 5.1 Phytochemicals identified in hydroalcoholic extract of licorice root by GC-MS

RT (min)	Name of the compound	Molecular formula*	Molecular weight* (g/mol)	Nature of the compound*	Bioactivity[†]
9.1	3-Hydroxy-3',4',5,7-tetramethoxyflavone	$C_{19}H_{18}O_7$	358.3	Flavone	Protector against lipid peroxidation, Antiviral, Anti proliferative
9.7	4H-1-Benzopyran-4-one,5,7-bis(acetyloxy)-2-[4-(acetyloxy)-3-methoxyphenyl]-3,6-dimethoxy-(jaceidin triacetate)	$C_{24}H_{22}O_{11}$	486.4	Flavone	Antibacterial
10.37	Undecane/ hendecane	$C_{11}H_{24}$	156.3	Alkane hydrocarbon	Not identified

* PubChem, Human Metabolome Database; [†]science.gov, Dr. Duke's Phytochemical and Ethnobotanical Database. RT: retention time.

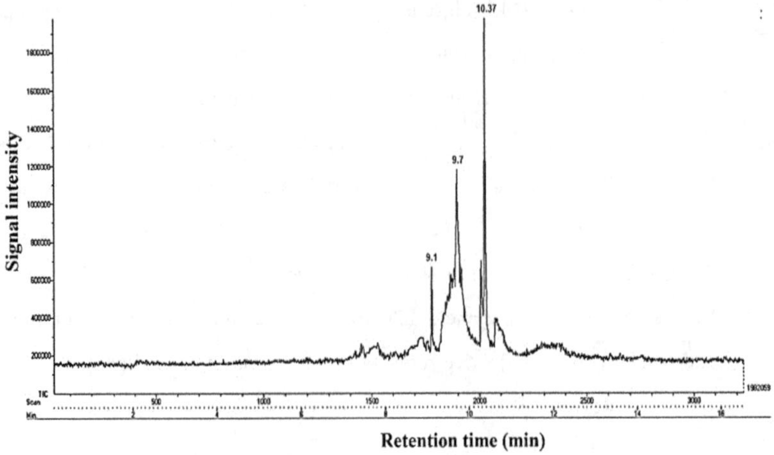

Figure 5.1 Ion chromatogram from the GC-MS analysis of hydroalcoholic extract of licorice root

Compounds were identified by matching the retention times with NIST database. RT 9.1= 3-Hydroxy-3',4',5,7-tetramethoxyflavone; RT 9.7= jaceidin triacetate; RT 10.37= undecane. RT: retention time in min.

5.1.2 HPLC analysis of hydroalcoholic extract of licorice root

HPLC is a chromatographic technique, used in phytochemistry and analytical chemistry to identify, quantify and purify the individual components of herbal extracts. Many studies have documented the use of HPLC for the characterization and quantification of secondary metabolites, and for the quality control assessment of medicinal plants [Thirumal Y,2017].

In this study, HPLC-UV chromatogram of HAELR flavonoids showed the presence of four major peaks at 270 nm with the retention times of 4.527, 11.310, 16.890 and 40.010 min **(Figure 5.2B)**. The peaks were identified as rutin, luteolin, thymoquinone and galangin at a concentration of 0.9 mg/g, 0.6 mg/g, 0.5 mg/g, and 1.3 mg/g, respectively. These flavonoids were confirmed by comparing their retention times with those of the corresponding standards **(Figure 5.2A)** and their estimated quantities were presented in **table 5.2**. Flavonoids have been proved scientifically to exhibit many biological properties like anti-oxidant, anti-mutagenic, antiinflammatory, and anti-viral effects, which can be developed as valuable therapeutic entities. Since ancient times, flavonoids or their respective preparations have been used to treat various human ailments, and their traditional usage has been continued throughout the ages. For example, plant-derived compounds like curcumin, resveratrol, and capsaicin were reported to inhibit inflammation by their action on the formation and activities of cytokines like IL-1β, IL-6, and TNF-α, and the suppression of COX-2, prostaglandins, through inflammatory pathways [Fürst R,2014].

Table 5.2 Quantitative estimation of phytochemicals in HAELR

Phytochemicals	Amount (mg/g of extract)
Rutin	0.957
Luteolin	0.626
Thymoquinone	0.574
Galangin	1.319
Glycyrrhizin	0.029

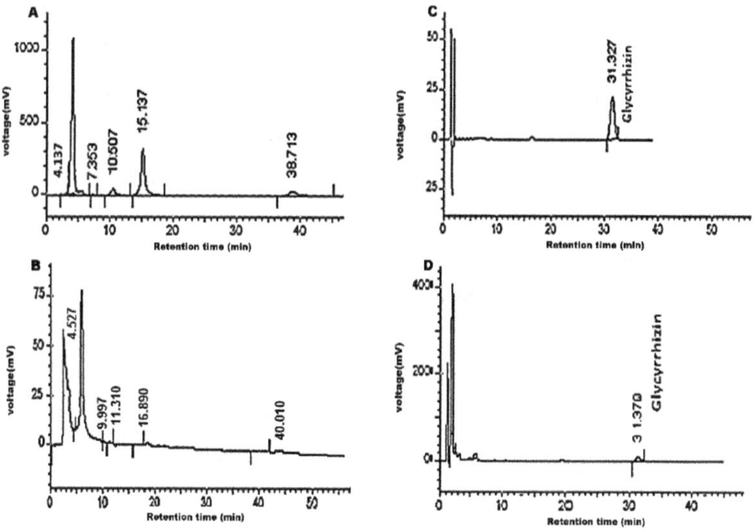

Figure 5.2 Chromatogram from the HPLC analysis of hydroalcoholic extract of licorice root

HPLC chromatogram of (A) flavanoid standards that were run, RT 4.137 =rutin; RT 10.507=luteolin; RT 15.137=thymoquinone; RT 38.713=galangin; (B) flavonoids that were detected in hydroalcoholic extract of licorice root, RT 4.527=Rutin; RT 11.310=luteolin; RT 16.890=thymoquinone; RT 40.010=galangin; (C) saponin standard run,which is glycyrrhizin; (D) saponins, that were detected in hydroalcoholic extract of licorice root. RT: retention time in min.

Figure 5.2D displays the HPLC-UV chromatogram of saponins of hydroalcoholic extract of licorice root. A peak was found at 254 nm with the retention time of 31.37 min. It was confirmed to be a saponin called glycyrrhizin, by matching the retention time and spectral characteristics with that of glycyrrhizin standard at different concentrations **(Figure 5.2C)**. Concentration of glycyrrhizin was calculated through a calibration graph and found to be 0.02 mg/g. Saponins are surface active glycosides produced mainly by plants. The hydrophilic sugar moeity and lipophilic aglycone moeity give saponins their amphiphilic nature, and they can easily penetrate into plasma membrane. This physicochemical property along with their wide range of biological activity makes saponins commercially significant in pharmaceutical industry. For example, ginseng saponins possess chemotherapeutic activity and are used in anticancer drug formulations, which were also patented [Huang D,2005] and HIV drugs like maturation inhibitors (PA — 457) are from pentacyclic triterpenoid saponin, betulinic acid [Bedoya LM,2018]. Many crude saponin extracts from *Camellia sinensis, Platycodon grandiflorum, Kalopanax pictus* were reported to show significant anti-inflammatory activity mostly by acting on COX-2 inflammatory pathway [Hassan HS,2012]. Many biological studies showed that different plant saponins have good antioxidant, antiviral, anti- cancer, antidepressant, anti-inflammatory, anti- carcinogenesis, hepatoprotective and neuroprotective activities. Diosgenin, the steroidal aglycone part obtained from saponin dioscin (present in *Dioscorea villosa* or wild yam), is the precursor for commercial production of steroids like cortisone, progesterone and pregnenolone [Kregiel D,2017].

With the presence these biologically important flavonoids and saponins confirmed from GCMS and HPLC analyses, HAELR could stand as a good alternative herbal drug.

5.2 Toxicity studies

5.2.1 Toxicity Estimation Software Tool (TEST)

Estimating the toxicity of drug is very essential to identify the possible harmful effects. It is a very basic and crucial step in drug design. Animal models were generally used for toxicity assessment. And, in vivo toxicity testing is time consuming, besides many ethical considerations. Hence, computational methods for toxicity estimation of drugs are considered important for chemical compounds. *Insilico* computational methods firstly analyze, simulate, visualize, to predict the toxicity of drugs.

TEST is one of the widely used computational tools to estimate toxicities from physical properties and molecular structure of drugs (called molecular descriptors). The required molecular descriptors can also be calculated using TEST itself [www.epa.gov]. TEST facilitates the toxicity estimation, without any need for external program. Drug to be evaluated is given as input, usually drawn using chemical sketcher window using molecular structure drawing tool or by entering as a structure text file, CAS number, SMILES string, or name. One can even import it from an existing database of structures as MDL molfile [Martin T,2016]. Once entered, the toxicity is automatically estimated using one of many Quantitative Structure Activity Relationship (QSAR) methodologies. Hierarchical clustering method is the default method in QSAR. Others include Single model method, nearest neighbor method, group contribution and consensus method [Muratov EN,2020]. Once the toxicity estimation calculations were being performed, a QSAR prediction report is generated automatically. Thus predicted oral rat LD_{50} for GZ using nearest neighbor method is is 88.39 mg/kg b. wt **(Table 5.3)**.

Table 5.3 Predicted Oral rat LD_{50} for GZ using Nearest neighbor method

Endpoint	Predicted value
Oralrat LD_{50} -Log10(mol/kg)	3.97
Oral rat LD_{50} mg/kg	88.39

The predicted LD_{50} value of GZ from TEST is 88.39 mg/kg b.wt

5.2.2 Acute and sub-chronic toxicity study

Safety assessment is of high priority for the human usage of plant extracts. Careful scientific validation of these herbal drugs regarding safety, identification of optimal therapeutic doses and efficacy in animal models is very essential for increased global acceptability and usage [Bhosale VV,2020]. Acute toxicity study, identifies the adverse effects of drug that result either from a single exposure or from multiple exposures in a short period of time (usually less than 24 hours). Chronic toxicity study identifies the adverse health effects of drug due to repeated exposures, often at lower levels, over a longer time period (months or years). Sub-chronic toxicity study identifies the toxicological effects of study-drug administered often, over a 90-day period [Yuet Ping K,2013]. Drugs intended for administration in chronic disease states may require, repeated dosing toxicological evaluation (as in sub-acute toxicity) because daily use may result in drug accumulation in the body with gradual effects on tissues and organs [Bariweni MW,2018].

5.2.2.1 LD_{50}

The adverse effects of the drug, if any, usually occur within 14 days of administration. LD_{50} is the one particular dose, that can kill 50% of study-animals under SOPs of drug administration. LD_{50} is a key parameter estimated in all acute toxicological studies [Erhirhie EO,2018]. The LD_{50} of HAELR calculated by karber method is 5000mg/kg b. wt as presented in **table 5.4**. The present acute toxicity study, performed by oral administration of HAELR to rats at different gradual doses (500,1000,2000,4000 and 5000 mg/kg b.wt.) did not show any mortality or toxicity during the treatment period.

From the observations of acute toxicity study, there is no death upto the test dose of 5000 mg/kg b.wt. in rats and all the doses tested are considered safe and nontoxic. When there are no observable signs of toxicity and mortality, even at final test dose (5000 mg/kg b. wt.) the LD_{50} of the test substance is said to be greater than 5,000 mg/kg b. wt [Shenbagam M,2011].

Table 5.4 Determination of LD_{50} value of HAELR by Karber's method

Group	HAELR (mg/kg b.wt)	Mortality
I	0	0
II	500	0
III	1000	0
IV	2000	0
V	4000	0
VI	5000	0

An upper dose level limit of 5,000 mg/kg b.wt. was introduced by OECD for substances whose expected LD_{50}values exceed 5,000 mg/kg b. wt [OECD,2002] [Erhirhie EO,2018]. With respect to these observations, determination of the precise LD_{50} would not be necessary and no further acute toxicity testing is required. Substances with LD_{50} at a dose range of 5000-15,000 mg/kg were practically non-toxic [Hayes AW,1996]. In the current study, HAELR was observed to be safe upto the dose level of 5000 mg/kg b. wt in rats. In an another acute toxicity study, ethanolic leaf extracts of Baccaurea ramiflora and Microcos paniculata were observed to be nontoxic and similar conclusions were made with respect to LD_{50} [Saha S,2017]. During HAELR chronic exposure (50, 100, 200, 400 and 500 mg/kg b.wt.) for 90days, there were no signs of adverse effects and no death occurred during this period.

5.2.2.2 General observations

For checking upon the morphological changes, general observations were made on appearance, behavior and physiology of rats subjected to acute and chronic exposure of HAELR and were presented in **table 5.5**.

Table 5.5 General observations on appearance, behavior and physiology of rats subjected to acute and chronic exposure of HAELR

Observations	Control	Acute oral exposure (5000 mg/kg b.wt of HAELR)	Chronic oral exposure (500 mg/kg b. wt of HAELR)
General physique	Normal	Normal	Normal
Changes in fur	No	No	No
Changes in skin	No	No	No
Swelling or lumps	Nil	Nil	Nil
Breathing difficulties	Nil	Nil	Nil
Dullness of eyes	Nil	Nil	Nil
Changes in eye color	No	No	No
Changes in teeth color	No	No	No
Digestion patterns	Normal	Normal	Normal
Biting	No	No	No
Licking	No	No	No
Self-mutilation	No	No	No
Disturbed sleep patterns	Nil	Nil	Nil
Aggression	Nil	Nil	Nil
Disturbed walk patterns	Nil	Nil	Nil
Abnormal posture	Nil	Nil	Nil
Hyperactivity	Nil	Nil	Nil
Lethargy	Nil	Observed initially	Observed initially
Tremors	Nil	Nil	Nil
Convulsions	Nil	Nil	Nil
Salivation	Nil	Nil	Nil
Lacrimation	Nil	Nil	Nil
Urination	Normal	Normal	Normal
Defecation	Normal	Normal	Normal
Coma	Nil	Nil	Nil
Death	Not observed	Not observed	Not observed

Although the major adverse effect is death in toxicity studies, non-lethal acute effects may occur as signs of toxicity depending on the drug being tested. To record these, visual signs of toxicity, morbidity and mortality were observed and is a key step in toxicity evaluation [Allen SL,2010]. Clinical observations like disturbances of walk patterns, abnormal posture, hyperactivity and lethargy including various other cage-side observations (**table 5.5**) were made, by close monitoring the animals every hour on the first day. From then, the observations were recorded once daily for 14-days in acute toxicity study. For the subchronic toxicity study, the observations were made twice daily for 90 days. In both acute and subchronic oral toxicity study, the animals did not show any visible sign of distress.

5.2.2.3 Body weight and organ weight

Any change, in body weight or weight of vital organs is a simple and sensitive index of toxicity and it can occur even in the absence of any morphological changes [Bouhrim M,2018].

A dose, which changes body weight by 10% or more, is generally toxic [Bhattacharjee A,2013]. The body weight of control and HAELR administered groups were monitored both in acute and chronic toxicity tests, as represented in **table.5.6** and were found to be similar without any significant changes. No significant changes were found even in the relative weight of the vital organs of HAELR- administered groups compared to control in both acute and chronic toxicity tests, as represented in **table.5.7**. Major objective of the organ weight analysis in toxicity study is to identify the target organs and drug related adverse effects [Nirogi R,2014]. Any increase in organ weight indicates, the occurrence of hypertrophy whereas, any decrease points out necrosis in the target organ. And a decrease in liver weight might be an evidence of toxicity [Ugwah-Oguejiofor CJ, 2019]. And is always suggested that organ weight findings must be interpreted with histopathological findings [Teo S,2002]. From the observations of organ weight, HAELR could be claimed safe for usage.

Table 5.6 Body weight of experimental rats subjected to acute and subchronic oral exposure to HAELR.

Acute toxicity study			Subchronic toxicity study		
No. of Days	Control	HAELR (5000mg/kg b.wt.)	No. of Days	Control	HAELR (500mg/kg b.wt.)
Day 0	191± 20.1	189 ± 18.7 NS	0 days	179 ± 17.3	171 ± 18.7 NS
Day 14	200 ± 20.7	197 ± 23. 6 NS	90days	227 ± 24.7	223 ± 28.9 NS

The body weight is expressed in grams, data represent mean ± standard deviation (SD), where n = 6. The results were analyzed statistically by comparing control vs HAELR in both studies. Changes were considered statistically significant when $p \leq 0.05$ and NS: non-significant.

Table 5.7 Relative organ weight of experimental rats subjected to acute and subchronic oral exposure to HAELR.

Organs	Control	HAELR (5000mg/kg b.wt.)	Control	HAELR (500mg/kg b.wt.)
Liver	3.51 ± 0.35	3.64 ± 0.40 NS	3.55±0.45	3.59 ± 0.38 NS
Kidney	1.02 ± 0.10	1.11 ± 0.13 NS	0.99±0.14	1.04 ± 0.11 NS
Heart	0.46 ± 0.05	0.49 ± 0.05 NS	0.50±0.06	0.47 ± 0.05 NS
Pancreas	0.72 ± 0.07	0.75 ± 0.08 NS	0.77±0.10	0.72 ± 0.08 NS
Brain	0.26 ± 0.02	0.29 ± 0.03 NS	0.38±0.05	0.31 ± 0.03 NS

The data represent mean ± standard deviation (SD), where n = 6. The results were analyzed statistically by comparing control vs HAELR in both studies. Changes were considered statistically significant when $p \leq 0.05$ and NS: non-significant. Relative organ weights were calculated as (organ weight (g)/body weight of animal on the day of sacrifice (g)) × 100.

5.2.2.4 Hematological parameters

Hematological parameters are considered as good indicators of the physiological changes and in turn health status of animals. These blood parameters can be altered by exposure to drugs especially medicinal plants [Christian AG,2017]. In the current investigation, all the studied hematological parameters like hemoglobin, RBC, WBC and platelet counts remained within physiological range after HAELR administration to rats during both acute and sub-chronic oral exposures. The non-significant activity of HAELR on RBC, shows that HAELR does not affect erythropoiesis and osmotic fragility of RBC. The WBC are the first line of defense which responds to infectious agents, inflammatory process or tissue injury [Olayode OA,2019]. High platelet at abnormal levels, may be indicative of haemostatic or thromboembolic disorder [Osei- Bimpong A,2012]. In this investigation, no significant changes were observed in WBC or platelet count of HAELR administered groups compared to respective controls in both acute and subchronic studies, as represented in **table.5.8**, further confirming the safety profile of HAELR.

Table 5.8 Hematological profile of experimental rats subjected to acute and subchronic oral exposure to HAELR.

Hematological parameter	Control	HAELR (5000mg/kg b.wt.)	Control	HAELR (500mg/kg b.wt.)
Haemoglobin(g %)	13.2 ± 1.34	12.9 ± 1.71 ^{NS}	13.0 ± 1.62	12.3 ± 1.35 ^{NS}
RBC Count (million/ mm^3)	5.7 ± 0.73	5.5 ± 0.61 ^{NS}	5.4 ± 0.77	5.0 ± 0.61 ^{NS}
WBC (cells/mm^3)	12760± 1429	12747 ± 1771^{NS}	12867± 1930	12859 ±1413 ^{NS}
Platelet(lakhs/mm^3)	1.9 ± 0.2	1.6 ± 0.17^{NS}	1.2 ± 0.13	1.0 ± 0.14^{NS}

The data represent mean ± standard deviation (SD), where n = 6. The results were analyzed statistically by comparing control vs HAELR in both studies. Changes were considered statistically significant when $p \leq 0.05$ and NS: non-significant.

5.2.2.5 Biochemical parameters

Functional liver and kidney are crucial for the survival of animals. Their functional status can be determined by serum biochemical analysis, which plays a key role in the toxicological evaluation of drugs. Serum AST, ALT and ALP activity levels are the markers of functional status of liver and their levels indicate any injury caused by the administration of test drugs [McGill MR,2016]. Raised levels of these liver enzymes indicates the presence of hepatocellular toxicity whereas decreased levels may indicate enzyme inhibition. Compared to AST and ALP, ALT is the better sensitive marker of liver damage or toxicity, since AST can also be abundantly found in kidneys, testes, cardiac and skeletal muscles [Ugwah-Oguejiofor CJ,2019]. Activities of ALT, AST and ALP in various experimental rats subjected to acute and chronic oral exposure to HAELR were represented in **table.5.9** and **table.5.12** respectively. And there observed no significant changes in the levels of these liver markers after HAELR administration.

Table 5.9 Activities of ALT, AST and ALP in various experimental rats subjected to acute oral exposure to HAELR.

HAELR (mg/kg b.wt.)	ALT (IU/L)	AST (IU/L)	ALP (IU/L)
Control (0)	21.87 ±2.66	20.49 ± 2.76	109.72± 15.47
500	20.32 ± 2.54 NS	19.39±2.9 NS	109.38 ±15.31 NS
1000	20.68 ± 2.89 NS	19.75 ± 2.90 NS	109.3 ± 12.1 NS
2000	21.7 ± 2.64 NS	20.2 ± 3.04 NS	109.43 ± 16.1 NS
4000	21.9 ±3.0 NS	20.5 ± 2.25 NS	109.8 ± 14.1 NS
5000	21.5 ±2.7 NS	20.38 ± 2.85 NS	108.7 ± 15.2 NS

The data represent mean ± standard deviation (SD), where n = 6. The results were analyzed statistically by comparing control vs HAELR. Changes were considered statistically significant when $p \leq 0.05$ and NS: non-significant.

Urea and creatinine levels in the blood are the markers of drug-induced renal damage [Fuchs TC,2011]. Increased serum LDH activity is considered as a marker of cellular necrosis and is used to assess the potential toxicity of drug [Kaja S,2017]. Levels of LDH, urea and creatinine along with blood glucose and protein levels in serum of various experimental rats subjected to acute and chronic oral exposure to HAELR were represented in **table.5.10** and **table.5.13** respectively.

Table 5.10 Serum levels of LDH, urea, creatinine, blood glucose and protein of various experimental rats subjected to acute oral exposure to HAELR

HAELR (mg/kg b.wt.)	LDH (IU/L)	Urea (mg/dL)	Creatinine (mg/dL)	Blood Glucose (mg/dL)	Protein (g/dL)
Control (0)	210.0 ± 23.1	23.9 ± 3.5	0.91 ± 0.10	73.5 ± 10.9	5.5±0.66
500	208.9±26.3 NS	23.3± 2.91 NS	0.93 ± 0.13 NS	72.1±9.5 NS	5.36±0.69 NS
1000	209.2±29.2 NS	23.7±3.19 NS	0.97 ±0.12 NS	72.4±9.05 NS	5.39±0.69 NS
2000	210.3±31.5 NS	23.9± 3.17 NS	0.99±0.11 NS	72.9±10.2 NS	5.35±0.80 NS
4000	212.4±26.1 NS	23.4± 3.36 NS	0.99 ± 0.12 NS	73.6±10.0 NS	5.29±0.66 NS
5000	213.3±30.5 NS	24.0±3.6 NS	0.96 ± 0.14 NS	73.4±8.8 NS	5.17±0.62 NS

The data represent mean ± standard deviation (SD), where n = 6. The results were analyzed statistically by comparing control vs HAELR. Changes were considered statistically significant when $p \leq 0.05$ and NS: non-significant.

Table 5.11 Serum levels of GSH and enzymatic antioxidants in experimental rats subjected to acute oral exposure to HAELR

HAELR (mg/kg b.wt.)	GSH (mg/dL)	GPx (U/L)	SOD (U/L)	CAT (U/L)
Control (0)	210.3 ± 29.6	23.7 ± 3.3	181.8 ± 26.1	0.311 ± 0.03
500	210.1 ± 28.3 ^{NS}	23.9 ± 3.5^{NS}	180.3 ± 25.2 ^{NS}	0.317 ± 0.04 ^{NS}
1000	209.4 ± 31.41 ^{NS}	24.6 ± 3.61 ^{NS}	182.1 ± 27.1 ^{NS}	0.316 ± 0.03 ^{NS}
2000	209.0 ± 30.9 ^{NS}	25.1 ± 3.63 ^{NS}	185.7 ± 25.6 ^{NS}	0.320 ± 0.03 ^{NS}
4000	209.8 ± 25.1 ^{NS}	25.9 ± 2.83 ^{NS}	185.7 ± 24.6 ^{NS}	0.323±0.037 ^{NS}
5000	211.2 ± 29.5 ^{NS}	26.2 ± 3.01 ^{NS}	185.4 ± 23.3 ^{NS}	0.325±0.036 ^{NS}

The data represent mean ± standard deviation (SD), where n = 6. The results were analyzed statistically by comparing control vs HAELR. Changes were considered statistically significant when $p \leq 0.05$ and NS: non-significant.

Table 5.12 Levels of ALT, AST, ALP in serum of various experimental rats subjected to sub-chronic (90-day) repeated oral dose of HAELR.

HAELR (mg/kg b.wt.)	ALT (IU/L)	AST (IU/L)	ALP (IU/L)
Control (0)	26.7±3.07	23.2±2.43	24.4±3.66
50	25.8±2.70^{NS}	23.5±2.89 ^{NS}	24.0±2.80 ^{NS}
100	26.2±2.85^{NS}	22.4±2.97 ^{NS}	23.5±3.12^{NS}
200	26.5±3.97 ^{NS}	24.2±2.90 ^{NS}	25.0±3.75 ^{NS}
400	26.5±3.16 ^{NS}	24.9±3.38 ^{NS}	25.9±3.65^{NS}
500	27.9±2.87 ^{NS}	25.1±2.88^{NS}	25.6±3.40^{NS}

The data represent mean ± standard deviation (SD), where n = 6. The results were analyzed statistically by comparing control vs HAELR. Changes were considered statistically significant when $p \leq 0.05$ and NS: non-significant.

Table 5.13 Levels of blood glucose and levels of LDH, urea, creatinine, protein in serum of various experimental rats subjected to sub-chronic (90-day) oral dose of HAELR.

HAELR (mg/kg b.wt.)	LDH (IU/L)	Urea (mg/dL)	Creatinine (mg/dL)	Blood glucose (mg/dL)	Serum Protein (g/dL)
Control(0)	205.9±22.8	20.9±3.13	0.58±0.064	92.4±11.0	3.49±0.36
50	205.2±27.9 NS	20.6±2.59NS	0.62±0.080NS	90.7±10.8 NS	3.45±0.34NS
100	206.3±27.85NS	19.9±2.98 NS	0.64±0.072 NS	91.1±11.6NS	3.51±0.47 NS
200	209.5±28.49NS	20.7±2.91NS	0.65±0.075 NS	91.9±12.4 NS	3.53±0.39 NS
400	209.9±28.75NS	21.3±2.55 NS	0.67±0.081 NS	92.8±13.5 NS	3.57±0.53 NS
500	210.4±31.34NS	21.8±2.96 NS	0.68±0.092 NS	91.5±13.3 NS	3.68±0.48 NS

The data represent mean ± standard deviation (SD), where n = 6. The results were analyzed statistically by comparing control vs HAELR. Changes were considered statistically significant when $p \leq 0.05$ and NS: non-significant.

The level of non-enzyme antioxidant GSH, and the levels of antioxidant enzymes like GPx, SOD and CAT, in various experimental rats subjected to acute and chronic oral exposure to HAELR were represented in **table.5.11** and **table.5.14** respectively. These are the indicators of status of oxidative stress, caused by the drug studied generally during toxicological studies [Ejeh SA,2019].

Table 5.14 Levels of antioxidants-GSH, GPx, SOD and CAT in serum of various experimental rats subjected to sub-chronic (90-day), oral dose of HAELR

HAELR (mg/kg b.wt.)	GSH (mg/dL)	GPx (U/L)	SOD (U/L)	CAT (U/L)
Control (0)	229.8 ± 30.56	25.9 ± 2.61	181.9 ± 25.6	0.262±0.029
50	229.5 ± 32.35 NS	26.2 ± 3.45 NS	181.7 ± 22.7 NS	0.260±0.035 NS
100	229.7 ± 32.3 NS	26.5 ± 3.60 NS	181.4 ± 22.9 NS	0.263±0.033 NS
200	229.1 ± 23.1 NS	26.8 ± 3.40 NS	182.3 ± 26.7 NS	0.264±0.033 NS
400	229.6 ± 25.0 NS	26.9 ± 2.93 NS	185.1 ± 23.3 NS	0.267 ± 0.027 NS
500	230.2 ± 23.7 NS	27.3 ± 2.86 NS	186.6 ± 27.9 NS	0.268 ± 0.028 NS

The data represent mean ± standard deviation (SD), where n = 6. The results were analyzed statistically by comparing control vs HAELR. Changes were considered statistically significant when $p \leq 0.05$ and NS: non-significant.

In the acute oral toxicity and sub-chronic oral toxicity, these serum measurements of liver markers, markers of damage to other vital organs (heart, kidney) and antioxidants in the HAELR administered groups did not show any significant difference from that of the control rats proving the non-toxic nature of HAELR. The observations of the current toxicity study are similar to another study where GutGard^{TM}, a standardized root extract from *Glycyrrhiza glabra* was analyzed for toxicity effects and shown safe upto 5000mg/kg b.wt. in rats [Raveendra KR,2012].

5.2.2.6 Histological studies

Histological examination is major criterion and gold standard for toxicology studies on animals and various observations can be made regarding target organs of drug toxicity [Fuchs TC,2011]. At the end of the respective study periods in both acute and subchronic oral toxicity studies, the vital organs like liver, kidney, heart, pancreas and brain were subjected to histopathological evaluation. Tissue sections of vital organs from the high dose-administered groups of acute (5000mg/kg b.wt.) and sub-chronic toxicity study (500mg/kg b.wt.) were represented in **figure 5.3** and **figure 5.4**. The photomicrograph of (A) liver showing normal tissue architecture with central vein, (B) kidney showing normal tissue architecture with prominent normal glomeruli (C) heart showing normal structure with cardiac myocytes (D) pancreas showing normal acinar and islets of Langerhans cells without any necrosis or edema (E) brain showing normal cerebral cortex area without any pathological deposits (H & E, 400x). Observations indicated normal morphological features and no alterations were found in the tissue architecture of the vital organs of HAELR administered groups compared to respective controls in both acute and subchronic toxicity studies. These histopathological observations supported the biochemical investigations of the study, confirming the safety of HAELR.

Figure 5.3(A-E): Effect of HAELR (5000mg/kg b.wt.) on liver, kidney, heart, pancreas and brain tissues-A histological photomicrograph

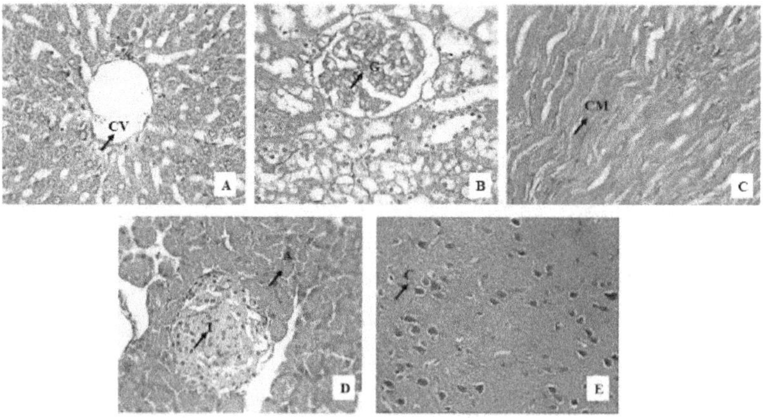

Note- Photomicrograph (H&E stained,400X magnification) of (A)Liver (B)Kidney (C)Heart (D)Pancreas (E)Brain

CV: central vein; G: glomerulus; CM: cardiac myocytes; A: acinar cell; I: islets of Langerhans; C: cerebral cortex.

Figure 5.4 (A-E): Effect of HAELR (500mg/kg b.wt.) on liver, kidney, heart, pancreas and brain tissues-A histological photomicrograph

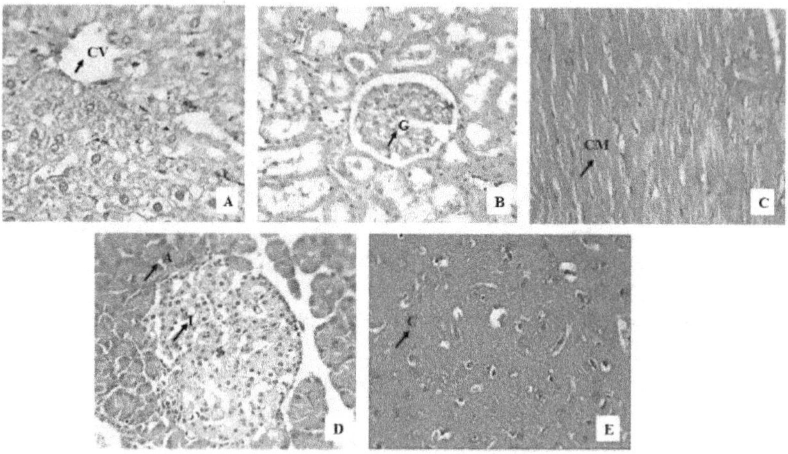

Note- Photomicrograph (H&E stained,400X magnification) of (A)Liver (B)Kidney (C)Heart (D)Pancreas (E)Brain

CV: central vein; G: glomerulus; CM: cardiac myocytes; A: acinar cell; I: islets of Langerhans; C: cerebral cortex.

5.3 Dose-response study

A dose-response study is a preliminary study, where different doses of a drug are tested against each other, to find out a single effective and least harmful dose. To find out the optimal therapeutic dose of HAELR/GZ against alcohol-cerulein induced pancreatitis, an initial dose-finding study was carried out. Rats were coadministered with different concentrations of HAELR (25,50,100 and 200 mg/kg b. wt) or GZ (2.5, 5, 10 and 20 mg/kg body wt). The levels of pancreatic enzyme markers (lipase and amylase) and inflammatory markers (MPO, Caspase-1, IL-1 β and IL-18) **(Table 5.15** to **Table 5.18)** were determined during the study. An optimal dose of 100mg/kg b. wt of HAELR and 10 mg/kg b. wt of GZ, which were shown to exhibit effective pancreato-protective activity, were chosen for all the further investigations.

Table 5.15 Dose response study - Serum levels of pancreatic marker enzymes in various experimental rats administered different doses of HAELR.

Pancreatic marker enzymes	Control	HAELR control	EtOH+ Cer	EtOH + Cer + HAELR (25mg/ kg b.wt.)	EtOH +Cer +HAELR (50mg/kg b.wt.)	EtOH + Cer +HAELR (100mg/kg b.wt.)	EtOH + Cer +HAELR (200mg/kg b.wt.)
Lipase (IU/L)	1643 ± 240	1640 ± 229 ^{NS}	2951 ± 344*	2520 ± 315*	2200± 291*	1750± 321.0**	1703 ± 358^{NS}
Amylase (IU/L)	127 ± 18.9	123 ± 14.8 ^{NS}	201± 30.1*	170 ± 20.6 *	150 ± 21.2 *	132 ± 18.7*	130 ± 13.9^{NS}

Data were analysed by one-way ANOVA followed by post-hoc Bonferroni test. Values are expressed as mean ± S.D. of six rats in each group. Statistical significance was calculated by comparing control vs. HAELR control, control vs. EtOH + Cer, EtOH + Cer vs. EtOH + Cer + HAELR, EtOH + Cer+ HAELR (25mg/kg) vs EtOH + Cer+ HAELR (50mg/kg b.wt), EtOH + Cer+ HAELR (50mg/kg) vs EtOH + Cer+ HAELR (100mg/kg b.wt), EtOH + Cer+ HAELR (100mg/kg) vs EtOH + Cer+ HAELR (200mg/kg b.wt), * $P < 0.05$; ** $P < 0.01$; NS: non-significant.

Table 5.16 Dose response study - Levels of serum inflammatory markers and pancreatic MPO activity in various experimental rats administered different doses of HAELR.

Group	MPO (U/mg protein)	Caspase-1 (pg/ml)	IL-1 β(pg/ml)	IL-18(pg/ml)
Control	5.7 ± 0.63	23.3 ± 3.4	16.5 ± 1.80	195.6±29.3
HAELR control	5.3 ± 0.67 NS	22.9 ± 2.5 NS	16.0±2.3 NS	210.2±31 NS
EtOH + Cer	11.5 ± 1.3*	45.2 ± 5.2*	37.8±4.1*	356.4±43*
EtOH + Cer+ HAELR (25mg/kg b.wt.)	10.0 ± 1.23 *	38.7 ± 4.0 *	29.5±4.4 **	306.2±42.5 *
EtOH + Cer+ HAELR (50mg/kg b.wt.)	8.09 ± 1.05**	33.4 ± 3.9 **	20.7±3.1 **	260.3±35.7 *
EtOH + Cer+ HAELR (100mg/kg b.wt.)	5.84± 0.8**	25.2 ± 2.7**	17.3±2.4*	219.1±31.1*
EtOH + Cer+ HAELR (200mg/kg b.wt.)	5.81 ± 0.6 NS	24.9 ± 2.5 NS	17.0±2.5 NS	213.6±30.2 NS

Data were analysed by one-way ANOVA followed by post-hoc Bonferroni test. Values are expressed as mean ± S.D. of six rats in each group. Statistical significance was calculated by comparing control vs. HAELR control, control vs. EtOH + Cer, EtOH + Cer vs. EtOH + Cer + HAELR, EtOH + Cer+ HAELR (25mg/kg) vs EtOH + Cer+ HAELR (50mg/kg b.wt), EtOH + Cer+ HAELR (50mg/kg) vs EtOH + Cer+ HAELR (100mg/kg b.wt), EtOH + Cer+ HAELR (100mg/kg) vs EtOH + Cer+ HAELR (200mg/kg b.wt), * P <0.05; ** P <0.01; NS: non-significant.

Table 5.17 Dose response study - Serum levels of pancreatic marker enzymes in various experimental rats administered different doses of GZ.

Pancreatic marker enzymes	Control	GZ control	EtOH+ Cer	EtOH + Cer +GZ (2.5mg/kg b.wt.)	EtOH + Cer +GZ (5 mg/kg b.wt.)	EtOH + Cer +GZ (10mg/kg b.wt.)	EtOH + Cer +GZ (20mg/kg b.wt.)
Lipase (IU/L)	1749 ± 180	1736 ± 208 NS	2997 ± 401*	2497 ± 347*	2142± 306*	1709± 251.0**	1699 ± 237NS
Amylase (IU/L)	131± 15.8	129 ± 17NS	212± 28.7*	177 ± 25 *	153± 22.5 *	134 ± 20*	131 ± 19.5NS

Data were analysed by one-way ANOVA followed by post-hoc Bonferroni test. Values are expressed as mean ± S.D. of six rats in each group. Statistical significance was calculated by comparing control vs. GZ control, control vs. EtOH + Cer, EtOH + Cer vs. EtOH + Cer + GZ, EtOH + Cer+ GZ (2.5mg/kg) vs EtOH + Cer+ GZ (5mg/kg b.wt), EtOH + Cer+ GZ (5mg/kg) vs EtOH + Cer+ GZ (10mg/kg b.wt), EtOH + Cer+ GZ (10mg/kg) vs EtOH + Cer+ GZ (20mg/kg b.wt), * P <0.05; ** P <0.01; NS: non-significant.

Table 5.18 Dose response study - Levels of serum inflammatory markers and pancreatic MPO activity in various experimental rats administered different doses of GZ.

Group	MPO(U/mg protein)	Caspase-1 (pg/ml)	IL-1 β(pg/ml)	IL-18(pg/ml)
Control	5.9± 0.60	23.5 ± 2.63	16.7± 2.03	200 ±26.4
GZ Control	5.8 ± 0.63^{NS}	23.1 ± 2.74^{NS}	16.9±2.18 ^{NS}	203.9±28.1 ^{NS}
EtOH + Cer	12.7 ± 1.44*	45.5± 5.64*	38.5±5.15*	360.7±49.4*
EtOH + Cer + GZ (2.5mg/kg b.wt.)	11.3 ± 1.31 *	39 ± 4.91*	30.4±4.13 **	310.3±41.8 *
EtOH + Cer + GZ (5mg/kg b.wt.)	9.2 ± 1.12 **	32.8 ± 4.32**	21.3±2.81 **	264.5±36.7 *
EtOH + Cer + GZ (10mg/kg b.wt.)	6.92± 0.85**	26.7 ± 3.57**	18.7±2.69*	223.8±31.7*
EtOH + Cer + GZ (20mg/kg b.wt.)	6.97± 0.87 ^{NS}	25.3± 3.41 ^{NS}	18.0±2.62 ^{NS}	218.9±32.6 ^{NS}

Data were analysed by one-way ANOVA followed by post-hoc Bonferroni test. Values are expressed as mean ± S.D. of six rats in each group. Statistical significance was calculated by comparing control vs. GZ control, control vs. EtOH + Cer, EtOH + Cer vs. EtOH + Cer + GZ, EtOH + Cer+ GZ (2.5mg/kg) vs EtOH + Cer+ GZ (5mg/kg b.wt), EtOH + Cer+ GZ (5mg/kg) vs EtOH + Cer+ GZ (10mg/kg b.wt), EtOH + Cer+ GZ (10mg/kg) vs EtOH + Cer+ GZ (20mg/kg b.wt), * *P* <0.05; ** *P* <0.01; NS: non-significant.

In a similar study, dose response (12.5,25 and 50 mg/kg) of oral antiulcer activity of, Glycyrrhiza glabra root extract, was determined to find out the optimum effective dose on gastric mucosal injury in rats [Mukherjee M,2010].

5.4 Therapeutic efficacy of HAELR and GZ

5.4.1 Effect of HAELR and GZ on pancreatic marker enzymes

The enzyme markers of EtOH and Cer-induced pancreatic injury are lipase and amylase activities, which are generally monitored in serum [Frulloni *et al.*, 2005]. Under physiological conditions, pancreatic digestive enzymes are synthesized in ER of pancreatic acinar cells, are transported as inactive pro-enzymes and gets activated only in the small intestine. Accurate protein processing by ER is extremely important, to avoid any premature activation of pancreatic enzymes inside acinar cells itself. Cytosolic calcium concentration and calcium release from ER, in response to hormonal stimuli is a signaling mechanism for this process. Alcoholic metabolites like FAEE and other fatty acids, along with Cer were shown to induce gradual release of calcium from ER, creating calcium store depletion leading to pathological calcium signaling patterns [Criddle 2006]. It can induce premature activation of pancreatic enzymes and subsequent pancreatic tissue destruction. Thus injured pancreatic acini, facilitate the release of pancreatic enzymes into the blood stream.

Both serum lipase and amylase levels were increased in pancreatitis-induced rats. These enzyme levels were reverted towards normal in rats, coadministered HAELR or GZ, highlighting their pancreato-protective effect as represented in **table 5.19**. In a previous study, it has been reported that increased serum amylase and lipase during pancreatitis, was significantly reduced by a traditional Iranian drug from *Echium amoenum* [Abed A, 2012].

Table 5.19 Effect of HAELR/GZ on the activity levels of pancreatitis marker levels in serum of various experimental rats

Groups	Lipase (IU/L)	Amylase (IU/L)
Control	1.74±0.22	1 831.21±218.01
HAELR Control	1.68±0.18 NS	1 715.02±223.82 NS
GZ Control	1.66±1.24 NS	1709±204 NS
EtOH + Cer	4.17±0.40*	3 872.48±398.49*
EtOH + Cer + HAELR	2.28±0.29*	2 298.79±264.29*
EtOH + Cer + GZ	3.23±0.35*	2400±315*

Data, analysed by one-way ANOVA followed by post-hoc Bonferroni test.Values, represented as Mean±SD and n=6 rats in each group. Statistical significance was then calculated by comparing control vs. HAELR control, control vs.GZ control, control vs. EtOH+Cer, EtOH+Cer vs. EtOH+Cer+HAELR and EtOH+Cer vs. EtOH+ Cer+GZ. *p represents 0.000, NS represents non-significant.

5.4.2 Effect of HAELR and GZ on oxidative stress

Chronic oxidative stress plays a pathophysiological role in CP, worsening, clinical symptoms. Overall, oxidative stress in pancreas is as a result of overproduction of ROS during xenobiotic metabolism. Pancreatic mitochondria produce most of the adenosine triphosphate (ATP) in mammalian cells. Substrates, when gets oxidized through mitochondrial respiratory chain, results in NADH formation along with ATP. Production of ATP is inevitably associated with the production of ROS. ROS are highly reactive molecules generated as metabolic by-products during ATP synthesis, which takes place at major sites like complex- I and complex-III of ETC. Ethanol, when converted to acetaldehyde by ADH and to acetate by ALDH, one molecule of NADH is produced in every reaction, supplying more reducing equivalents (NADH) to mitochondria. These excess reducing equivalents facilitates the transfer of electrons to molecular oxygen propagating the cycle of excess ROS generation. Shalbueva *et al.* reported that ethanol treatment led to a decrease in the NAD^+/NADH ratio in isolated pancreatic acinar cells [Shalbueva N,2013]. So ethanol increases redox pressure in mitochondria through NADH, promoting the formation of ROS. The pathologic effect of cerulein in stimulating mitochondrial ROS production was reported to be by abnormal calcium signaling [Kim H,2008]. ROS were known to cause potential damage to cellular constituents. Physiologically, ROS are safely neutralized by the antioxidant defense mechanisms both inside and outside the mitochondria. In pancreatitis, infiltrating inflammatory cells, ethanol metabolism through CYP2E1, NADPH oxidase of PSCs and xanthine oxidase released by damaged pancreas could act as sources of intracellular ROS production [Kikuta K,2004] [Masamune A,2008] [Folch E, 1998]. So, pancreatic acinar cells are prone to tremendous oxidative stress under the influence of alcohol and cerulein.

The attenuation of oxidative stress by HAELR/GZ in the study, is evidenced by the levels of total peroxide content, TAC and OSI as presented in **table 5.20**. Enzymatic (SOD, CAT, GPx) and non-enzymatic free radical scavengers (GSH) work in coordination in cells, against free radicals to maintain ideal redox status in living cells. But, when the produced ROS levels overcome the cellular antioxidant defense systems, the equilibrium turns towards ROS formation as noted in rats administered ethanol and cerulein. After co-administration with HAELR or GZ, the enzyme levels were reverted towards normal, highlighting amelioration of oxidative stress by these test drugs as shown in **table 5.21**.

Table 5.20 Effect of HAELR/GZ on oxidative stress markers in plasma of experimental rats

Group	Total peroxide (TP)(mmol/ml)	TAC (mmol trolox eq./L)	OSI(TP/TAC)
Control	172.3±20.8	332.4±44.54	0.51±0.05
HAELR Control	171.4±24.3 NS	330.9±45.9 NS	0.49±0.06 NS
GZ control	169.8±23.2 NS	319.9±45.10 NS	0.53±0.06NS
EtOH + Cer	287.5±34.2*	227.1±29.52*	1.26±0.17*
EtOH+Cerulein+HAELR	206.1±25.7*	300.1±42.6*	0.79±0.08*
EtOH +Cer+GZ	194.0±21.7*	302.5±33.95*	0.64±0.12*

Data, analysed by one-way ANOVA followed by post-hoc Bonferroni test. Values, represented as Mean±SD and n=6 rats in each group. Statistical significance was then calculated by comparing control vs. HAELR control, control vs. GZ control, control vs. EtOH+Cer, EtOH+Cer vs. EtOH+Cer+HAELR and EtOH+Cer vs. EtOH+Cer+GZ. *p represents 0.000, NS represents non-significant.

Table 5.21 Effect of HAELR/GZ on antioxidant levels in the pancreas of experimental animals.

Groups	GSH (mg/g protein)	GPx (nM GSH oxidized/min/ mg protein)	SOD (Units/mg protein)	CAT (μM of H_2O_2 consumed/min/mg protein)
Control	56.20±6.57	80.20±10.34	13.50±1.53	105.20±13.00
HAELR control	55.30±6.85 NS	79.80±9.57 NS	13.00±1.67 NS	103.60±11.95 NS
GZ control	54.1±6.17 NS	78.3±8.61 NS	13.17±1.61 NS	104.9±15.73 NS
EtOH +Cerulein	21.40±3.18*	48.80±6.99*	6.90±0.96*	70.90±10.45*
EtOH +Cerulein + HAELR	44.50±6.43*	68.20±8.72*	11.20±1.40*	97.40±10.90*
EtOH+Cer + GZ	41.9±5.8*	65.87±8.95*	10.34±1.65*	95.9±13.6*

Data, analysed by one-way ANOVA followed by post-hoc Bonferroni test. Values, represented as Mean±SD and n=6 rats in each group. Statistical significance was then calculated by comparing control vs. HAELR control, control vs. GZ control, control vs. EtOH+Cer, EtOH+Cer vs. EtOH+Cer+HAELR and EtOH+Cer vs. EtOH+ Cer+GZ. *p represents 0.000, NS represents non-significant.

GZ, at a dose of 50 mg/kg was previously shown to attenuate oxidative stress and inflammation by preserving antioxidant enzyme activities, in the lithium/pilocarpine-induced model of status epilepticus seizures [González-Reyes S,2016].

5.4.3 Effect of HAELR and GZ on lipid peroxidation

ROS are chemically reactive species and could always cause lipid peroxidation. The products of lipid peroxidation MDA and 4-HNE, are the reliable markers of lipid peroxidation. They indicate the ROS-dependent tissue damage and thus were monitored in the study [Kwiecien S,2014]. Increased levels of TBARS (MDA) and 4-HNE were observed in the pancreatitis induced rats, and these levels decreased significantly in rats coadministered either HAELR/GZ as shown in **table 5.22**. The results brought to light that, HAELR/GZ improved the antioxidant status and decreased the incidence of free radical-induced pancreatic injury.

Table 5.22 Effect of HAELR/GZ on lipid peroxidation products in the pancreas of experimental animals

Groups	TBARS (MDA) (nM/mg protein)	4-HNE (µM/g protein)
Control	29.80±3.14	1.98±0.22
HAELR control	30.70±3.77 ^{NS}	2.12±0.27 ^{NS}
GZ control	30.98±4.6 ^{NS}	2.0±0.29 ^{NS}
EtOH + Cerulein	51.10±5.57*	8.30±0.84*
EtOH + Cerulein + HAELR	33.90±4.17*	4.89±0.59*
EtOH + Cer + GZ	35.85.08*	5.25±0.65*

Data, analysed by one-way ANOVA followed by post-hoc Bonferroni test. Values, represented as Mean±SD and n=6 rats in each group. Statistical significance was then calculated by comparing control vs. HAELR control, control vs. GZ control, control vs. EtOH+Cer, EtOH+Cer vs. EtOH+Cer+HAELR and EtOH+Cer vs. EtOH+Cer+GZ. **p* represents 0.000, NS represents non-significant.

5.4.4 Effect of HAELR and GZ on inflammatory markers

Hallmark features of CP include acinar cell atrophy and chronic inflammation. In response to pre-disposing insults, injured pancreatic acinar cells trigger an inflammatory process by the release of inflammatory cytokines and chemokines, that mediate the recruitment and activation of circulating neutrophils and macrophages. Thus activated neutrophils, release excess pro-oxidants and cytotoxic agents, worsening the local damage in pancreas. As the inflammation advances, neutrophils transmigrate across endothelial cells and cause systemic inflammatory response syndrome, dysfunction of vital organs and, sometimes, to organ failure and death [Yang ZW,2015].

Degree of pancreatic inflammatory cell infiltration was measured in terms of tissue concentrations of MPO [Simsek O,2018]. MPO is one of the widely used pro-inflammatory biomarker, in various inflammatory diseases (like tuberculosis, asthma, rheumatoid arthritis, chronic hepatitis) and other major ailments (ischemic heart diseases and acute coronary syndrome). This enzyme is released into the extracellular medium by the neutrophils during inflammatory processes at the site of infection [Khan AA,2018]. Elevated MPO concentration was observed in pancreatitis-induced rats, mirroring the extent of tissue inflammation. MPO concentration decreased significantly in HAELR or GZ coadministered rats, indicating their anti-inflammatory potency as presented in **table 5.23**. Bioactive compounds like flavonoids and saponins in HAELR might have contributed to its anti-inflammatory properties.

Table 5.23 Effect of HAELR/GZ on Inflammatory markers in serum and pancreas.

Groups	MPO (Units/mg protein)	Caspase -1		IL-1 beta (pg/ml)	IL-18 (pg/ml)
		Serum (pg/ml)	Pancreas (pM/mg protein		
Control	2.93±0.33	12.3±1.76	12.5±1.41	14.9±1.65	190.3±30.03
HAELR control	2.77±0.32 NS	11.4±1.20 NS	11.3±1.38 NS	14.1±1.78 NS	201.2±25.50 NS
GZ control	2.8±0.34 NS	12.0±1.68 NS	12±1.72 NS	14.5±1.62 NS	196.8±24.2 NS
EtOH+Cerulein	5.04±0.69*	23.2±2.52*	48.8±5.27*	29.7±4.12*	345.5±42.10*
EtOH+ Cerulein +HAELR	3.49±0.52*	15.1±1.89*	21.2±2.54*	19.3±2.10*	219±29.78*
EtOH +Cerulein + GZ	3.78±0.53*	16.7±2.0*	21.9±2.69*	20.2±3.0*	230.6±34.3*

Data, analysed by one-way ANOVA followed by post-hoc Bonferroni test. Values, represented as Mean±SD and n=6 rats in each group. Statistical significance was then calculated by comparing control vs. HAELR control, control vs. GZ control, control vs. EtOH+Cer, EtOH+Cer vs. EtOH+Cer+HAELR and EtOH+Cer vs. EtOH+Cer+GZ. *p represents 0.000, NS represents non-significance.

ROS also triggers many inflammatory processes. Yu *et al.* has shown that cerulein enhances ROS production, activates NF-κB, and its subsequent cytokine expression, suggesting a probable causal relationship, between ROS and inflammatory cytokines in the pancreatic acinar cells. It has also been reported that, these alterations are inhibited by endogenous antioxidants [Yu JH,2002]. ROS is a proven chemoattractant for many inflammatory cells [Kim H,2008].

Caspase-1 is the extensively monitored inflammatory caspase, which gets activated through inflammasome assembly. It initiates the inflammatory responses through the activation of pro-inflammatory cytokines like interleukin-1β and interleukin-18. Role of inflammasomes and caspase-1 is studied widely, in the development and progression of many inflammation-induced noncommunicable diseases like obesity, diabetes, cardiovascular diseases, cancers and chronic respiratory diseases [Molla MD,2020]. Among the major IL1 cytokines, IL1β mediates pancreatic inflammation actively. IL1β is known to be transcribed by monocytes, macrophages, and dendritic cells as a consequence of TLR activation by PAMPs or by other cytokines TNFα, IL18, IL1α or IL1β itself. IL1β is generally not present in healthy cells [Dinarello CA,1987]. IL18 is expressed by macrophages, epithelial cells and dendritic cells and is usually stored in the cytoplasm. Serum levels of IL18 were reported to be correlated with disease severity of pancreatitis in humans [Janiak A,2015].

Caspase-1, IL-1β and IL-18 also mediates pancreatic injury and inflammation and their serum levels gets altered after chronic ethanol exposure [Hoque R,2015]. Existing studies revealed that, enhanced levels of IL-1β and IL-18 induce CP [Marrache F,2008] [Schneider A,2006]. In the study, the serum levels of caspase-1, IL-1β and IL-18 were found increased significantly in pancreatitis-induced rats compared to control. HAELR/GZ co-administrations decreased the levels of these inflammatory markers towards normal, showing their ability to inhibit the production of active IL-1β and IL-18. Similar inactivation was shown to reduce the severity of pancreatitis [Ning JW,2017]. These observations draw special attention to highly potent anti-inflammatory nature of HAELR and GZ.

5.4.5 Effect of HAELR and GZ on NF-κB

The major event responsible for pancreatic inflammation is NF-κB activation. Sustained ER stress activates inflammatory pathways through chronic NF-κB activation in CP [Sah, 2014]. Many studies have shown ER stress, to downregulate IκBα, an inhibitor of NF-κB leading to NF-κB activation. EtOH also causes activation of NF-κB directly through the activation of protein kinase C in pancreatic acini [Gukovskaya, 2004]. Oxidative metabolism of ethanol to acetaldehyde by CYP2E1 produces excessive ROS which also activates ROS sensitive NF-κB [Apte MV,2016]. The activated NF-κB, triggers expression of pro-inflammatory cytokines and chemokines increasing the severity of pancreatitis. It has also been well documented that, inhibition of NF-κB improves pancreatic function [Huang, 2013]. An up-regulated mRNA expression of NF-κB was observed in pancreatitis-induced rats and, HAELR/GZ co-administrations were found to augment it significantly as represented in **figure 5.5**.

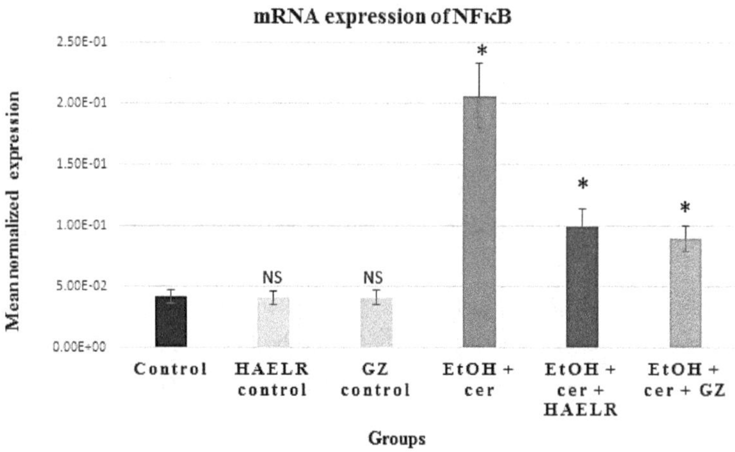

Figure 5.5 Gene expression analysis of NF-κB studied by qPCR indicating the effect of HAELR/GZ.

Mean normalized values were expressed as mean ± S.D and n=6. Statistical significance was calculated by means of one-way ANOVA and post-hoc Bonferroni test by comparing control and HAELR/ GZ control; control and EtOH + Cer; EtOH + Cer and EtOH + Cer + HAELR/ EtOH + Cer + GZ; * P represents 0.05; NS represents not significance.

The amelioration of NF-κB activation by HAELR and GZ might be due to the reduction of excessive ROS by both the test drugs, attributed to their excellent anti-oxidative nature.

5.4.6 Effect of HAELR and GZ on ER stress

The metabolism of ethanol in pancreas disturbs ER homeostasis, by causing accumulation of improperly folded proteins, leading to substantial activation of UPR and stress in ER. Acinar cells may be elicited to injury and death in the due course of disease [Criddle,2007]. Oxidative stress could be a probable mechanism behind the induction of pancreatic ER stress by EtOH. A study by Waldron *et al*, has reported that EtOH through its oxidative effect caused distortions in the structure of ER, promoting ER stress-related pathology in mouse pancreas. All these pathological changes are further aggravated in response to Cer [Waldron, 2018]. Chronic ER stress is well documented to be a primary cellular patho-mechanism of pancreatitis.

In this study, ER stress was investigated by monitoring the mRNA expressions of its UPR components-GRP78, ATF4, CHOP, XBP1. Protein processing in ER is executed by these chaperones. GRP78 is an abundant ER-specific chaperone belonging to HSP70 family and this protein inactivates other chaperones like PERK, IRE1 and ATF6, which relate ER stress to UPR stimulation. When unfolded proteins pile up, GRP78 leaves the three receptors leading to the stimulation of these receptors and triggering of respective UPR pathways. GRP78 is very sensitive to ER stress [Chaudhari N, 2014]. XBP1 is an active factor of transcription for the production of GRP78. Overexpression of mRNA level of XBP1 was documented previously in CP. Stimulation of IRE1/XBP1 pathway is a cellular stress response to re-establish ER protein processing [Sah, 2014]. ATF4 is involved in the transcription of genes needed to restore disturbed ER homeostasis and activates the genes encoding antioxidative stress responses. ATF4, also activates, genes responsible for the regulation of intracellular redox status and GSH synthesis. Elevated CHOP is related to uncontrolled inflammation as it regulates cytokine production and promotes increased number of inflammatory cells. CHOP also causes the production of interleukin-1 β by triggering caspase-1 through caspase-11, leading to inflammatory stress responses [Nishitoh, 2012]. Together, the UPR mechanisms alleviate ER stress to maintain ER homeostasis as represented in **figure 5.6**. It is very important for a functional acinar cell during both normal and diseased states. But if the ER stress is not rectified, persistent stimulation of the UPR takes place.

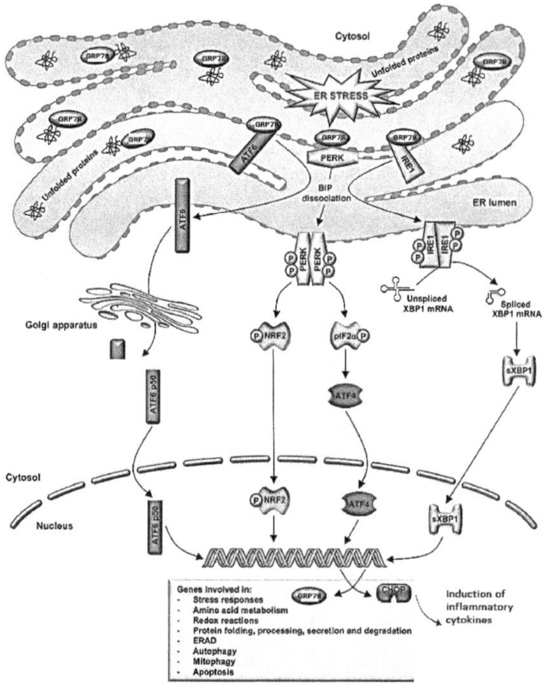

Figure 5.6 Role of UPR components in ER stress

(Source: https://www.frontiersin.org/articles/10.3389/fphys.2018.01744/full)

In the study, a sustained up-regulation of mRNA expressions of all the four UPR components-ATF4, CHOP, GRP78, and XBP1 was seen in pancreatitis-induced rats, which revealed the existence of persistent ER stress. HAELR/GZ co-administration significantly reduced the EtOH and Cer-induced ER stress as observed from downregulated expression of these genes in HAELR and GZ coadministered rats as presented in **figure 5.7 to figure 5.10**. The total cDNAs which has been amplified for the respective target genes subjected to agarose gel electrophoresis are shown in **figure 5.11**. Lugea *et al*, hypothesized that pancreas initiates this adaptive UPR to reduce the ER stress generated by alcohol [Lugea, 2015]. But when it is beyond the protective capacity of UPR, it progresses to CP. Our study highlighted the pancreas-protective effect of HAELR and GZ in EtOH and Cer-induced CP with UPR as a definitive target.

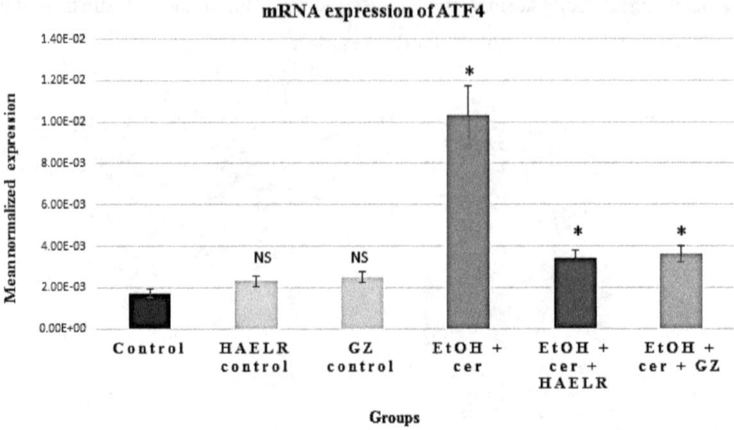

Figure 5.7 Gene expression analysis of ATF4 studied by qPCR indicating the effect of HAELR/GZ.

Mean normalized values were expressed as mean ± S.D and n=6. Statistical significance was calculated by means of one-way ANOVA and post-hoc Bonferroni test by comparing control and HAELR/ GZ control; control and EtOH + Cer; EtOH + Cer and EtOH + Cer + HAELR/ EtOH + Cer + GZ; * P represents 0.05; NS represents not significance.

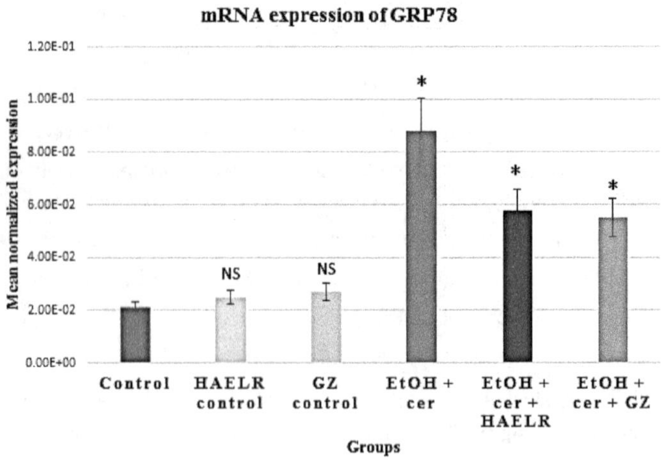

Figure 5.8 Gene expression analysis of GRP78 studied by qPCR indicating the effect of HAELR/GZ.

Mean normalized values were expressed as mean ± S.D and n=6. Statistical significance was calculated by means of one-way ANOVA and post-hoc Bonferroni test by comparing control and HAELR/ GZ control; control and EtOH + Cer; EtOH + Cer and EtOH + Cer + HAELR/ EtOH + Cer + GZ; * P represents 0.05; NS represents not significance.

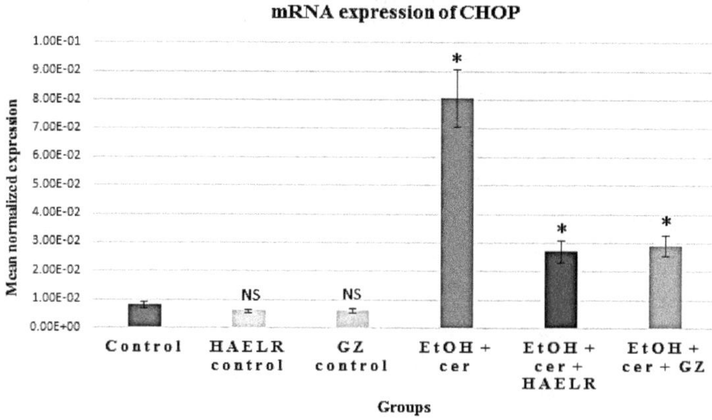

Figure 5.9 Gene expression analysis of CHOP studied by qPCR indicating the effect of HAELR/GZ.

Mean normalized values were expressed as mean ± S.D and n=6. Statistical significance was calculated by means of one-way ANOVA and post-hoc Bonferroni test by comparing control and HAELR/ GZ control; control and EtOH + Cer; EtOH + Cer and EtOH + Cer + HAELR/ EtOH + Cer + GZ; * P represents 0.05; NS represents not significance.

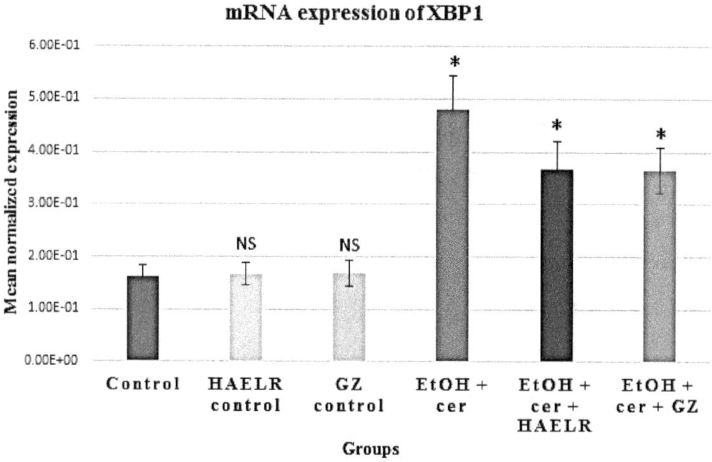

Figure 5.10 Gene expression analysis of XBP1 studied by qPCR indicating the effect of HAELR/GZ.

Mean normalized values were expressed as mean ± S.D and n=6. Statistical significance was calculated by means of one-way ANOVA and post-hoc Bonferroni test by comparing control and HAELR/ GZ control; control and EtOH + Cer; EtOH + Cer and EtOH + Cer + HAELR/ EtOH + Cer + GZ; * P represents 0.05; NS represents not significance.

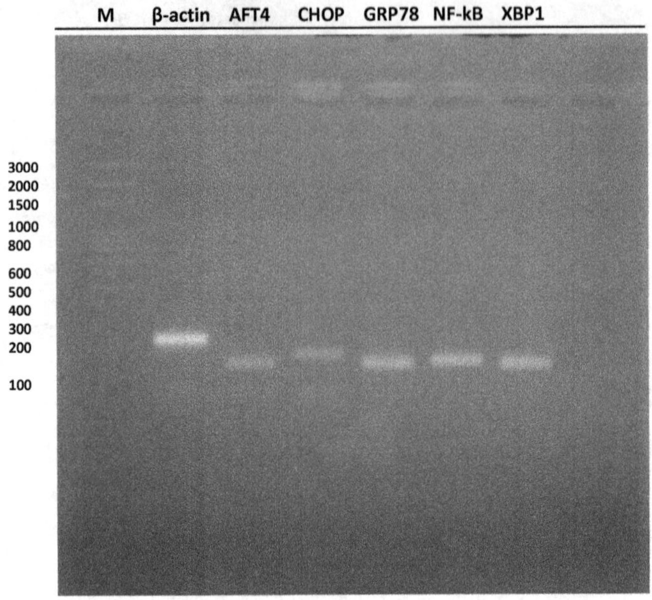

Figure 5.11: Agarose gel image of amplification products

5.4.7 Effect of HAELR/GZ on mitochondrial oxidative stress and $[Ca^{2+}]_m$.

Pancreatic acinar cells contain excess mitochondria as energy sources for the synthesis of digestive enzymes. Pancreatic mitochondria are more susceptible intracellular targets to EtOH-induced injury. Alcoholic metabolites disturb pancreatic mitochondrial functions and causes acinar cell death by aberrant calcium signaling [Clemens DL, 2014]. As the excess calcium released from ER, in response to alcoholic metabolites reaches pancreatic mitochondria, sustained elevation of mitochondrial calcium takes place. Mitochondrion is the major intracellular origin of ROS. Physiologically, many super oxides and hydrogen peroxides are formed during mitochondrial ETC. Mitochondrial ROS further promotes calcium release from nearby ER and increases $[Ca^{2+}]_m$ accumulation, initiating a positive feedback. Excessive release of calcium to mitochondria leads to calcium stimulated oxidative damage to mitochondria, failure of ATP production, energy deprivation and cellular necrosis [Cao and Kaufman, 2014]. Toxic accumulation of mitochondrial ROS is usually defended by GSH, GPx, SOD and CAT. To investigate the mitochondrial oxidative stress GSH, GPx, SOD and CAT levels were determined. Oxidative stress completely disrupts mitochondrial membrane, as shown by excess lipid peroxidation products like TBARS and 4-HNE, affecting permeability. A significant decrease in the levels of antioxidants accompanied by an increase in lipid peroxidation products was observed in pancreatitis-induced rats compared to control. HAELR/GZ co-administration improved these pathological changes as represented in **table 5.24**. Reduced activities of SOD and GPx have been reported to cause mitochondrial oxidative stress [Zang Q, 2007]. Disturbed mitochondrial function is one of the leading cause for the onset and progression of pancreatitis. It has been clear from the study results that, HAELR/GZ treatment can be a good strategy to target mitochondria, in order to locally scavenge ROS at their site of origin itself. Similarly, MitoQ and SKQ1 were shown to be effective against pancreatitis in a previous study, by acting as scavengers of ROS [Weniger ,2016] [Huang, 2015].

Table 5.24 Effect of HAELR/GZ treatment on the levels of mitochondrial oxidative markers, lipid peroxidation products and $[Ca^{2+}]_m$.

Group	GSH (mg/g protein)	Gpx (nM GSH oxidized/min/mg protein)	SOD (units/mg protein)	CAT (μ mol H_2O_2 consumed/ min/mg protein)	TBARS (nM/mg protein)	4-HNE (μM/g protein)	$[Ca^{2+}]_m$ (nM)
Control	4.8±0.61	122.3±16.38	6.9±0.70	5.1±0.57	8.6±1.075	0.040±0.006	91.63±11.08
HAELR control	4.73±0.62 ^{NS}	120.6±14.8 ^{NS}	6.71±0.77 ^{NS}	5.0±0.75 ^{NS}	9.0±1.3 ^{NS}	0.035±0.007 ^{NS}	93.0±12.3 ^{NS}
GZ control	4.6±0.60^{NS}	119.7±15.20^{NS}	6.7±0.73^{NS}	4.8±0.61^{NS}	9.2±1.104^{NS}	0.035±0.004^{NS}	93.7±11.99^{NS}
EtOH +Cer	2.7±0.39*	79.4±11.43*	3.6±0.42*	2.6±0.26*	13.1±1.89*	0.132±0.017*	168.9±20.09*
EtOH + Cerulein+ HAELR	4.2±0.47*	112±13.7*	5.7±0.80*	4.8±0.72*	11.0±1.5*	0.073±0.009*	90.2±11.1*
EtOH +Cer+ GZ	3.9±0.43*	109.3±14.20*	5.2±0.62*	4.0±0.48*	10.4±1.16*	0.067±0.007*	79.5±9.14*

Values represent mean ± S.D where n=6. Statistical significance was denoted through one-way ANOVA and post-hoc Bonferroni test by comparing control and HAELR control/GZ control; control and EtOH + Cer; EtOH + Cer and EtOH + Cer + HAELR/ EtOH + Cer + GZ; * $P < 0.05$; NS: not significant.

ER stress and mitochondrial oxidative stress are interlinked pathological events of CP mediated through calcium. To determine the [Ca $^{2+}$]$_m$ concentration, fura-2AM which is a membrane permeable, non-invasive, ratio metric indicator was used. It can accumulate to a variable extent when loaded onto mitochondrial isolates [Sheu and Sharma, 1999]. In this study, [Ca $^{2+}$]$_m$ concentration in pancreatitis-induced rats was found to be significantly higher than that of control and HAELR/GZ co-administration found to attenuate the increase as represented in **table 5.24**. Although a small increase in [Ca $^{2+}$]$_m$ concentrations boost up enzyme activity and subsequent ATP synthesis, excessive [Ca $^{2+}$]$_m$ load disable ATP synthesis [Brookes, 2004]. The results showed attenuation of [Ca $^{2+}$]$_m$ overload by HAELR and GZ. Odinokova IV *et al,* 2009 documented that, mitochondrial ROS levels and mitochondrial calcium regulates the functional capacity of acinar cells during pancreatitis. Their reports also pointed out that, stabilizing mitochondria against such functional loss may be a good approach to reduce the severity of pancreatitis. Mitochondrial cytochrome C is released under the influence of [Ca $^{2+}$]$_m$ over load and excess ROS . The loss of cytochrome C has been shown to inhibit the ETC leading to mitochondrial dysfunction [Odinokova, 2009].

5.4.8 Effect of HAELR/GZ on mitochondrial functions

Mitochondrial functional status was investigated through complex-1 activity in the isolated mitochondria. Complex-1 is reported to be severely affected in mitochondrial oxidative stress [Wu J,2015]. Early organ specific pancreatic mitochondrial dysfunction in Cer-induced pancreatitis was described by previous studies [Trumbeckaite S,2013]. Acetaldehyde, was found to destabilize the ETC and affects mitochondrial functioning [Manzo-Avalos and Saavedra-Molina, 2010]. In this study, marked decrease of mitochondrial complex-1 activity was observed in pancreatitis-induced rats, and it was found to be restored with HAELR/GZ co-administration as shown in **figure 5.12**. Mitochondrial compex-1 is positioned in the inner mitochondrial membrane, which is susceptible to lipid peroxidation. The formed 4-HNE has been demonstrated to produce HNE-protein adducts with complex-1, affecting its function. It was illustrated in mitochondrial isolates of diabetic rat kidney by Wu *et al* [Wu J, 2015]. Sun *et al* demonstrated that chronic alcohol feeding to rats, increases the 4-HNE levels in liver mitochondria leading to impaired functioning of respiratory complexes. The defective complexes of ETC can further exacerbate ROS generation in mitochondria [Sun Q, 2016]. The other physiological consequence of complex-1 impairment is, a decline in mitochondrial ATP production and energy deprivation. HAELR/ GZ co-administration maintained the activity of complex-1 and this might be by modulating 4-HNE level, by both the test drugs, underlining their protection against mitochondrial damage in CP.

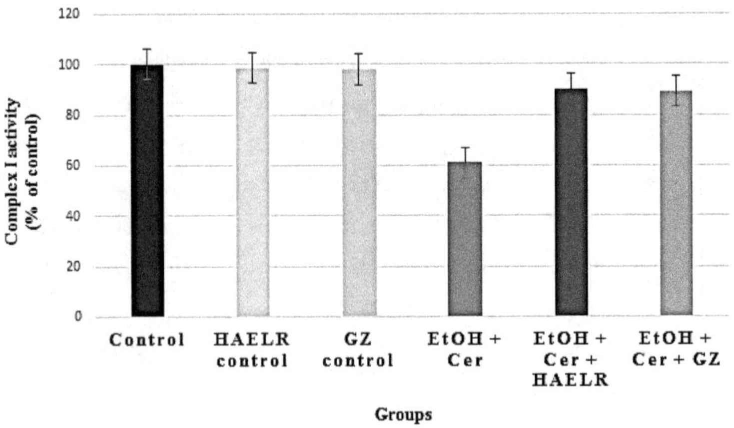

Figure 5.12 Mitochondrial ETC: Complex-1 activity

Complex-1 activity from mitochondrial isolates of various experimental groups indicating the attenuation of EtOH +Cer induced mitochondrial functional abnormality by HAELR and GZ. Values of HAELR control, GZ control, EtOH + Cer, EtOH + Cer + HAELR and EtOH + Cer + GZ were expressed as percentage activity of control.

In brief, high levels of calcium released from ER into pancreatic mitochondria causes calcium stimulated mitochondrial oxidative stress and subsequently complex-1 impairment. Dysfunctional mitochondria can harm pancreatic cells by cellular oxidative stress [Zhou, 2011]. An ROS-generating mitochondrion has also been shown to activate NLRP3 inflammasome complex. NLRP3 recognizes damage associated molecular patterns produced by damaged mitochondria, serves as a signaling platform for the activation of caspase-1 and release of pro-inflammatory cytokines like interleukin- 1β and interleukin-18. Mitochondria-induced NLRP3 inflammasome activation might be a probable reason for the frequent incidence of mitochondrial damage in various inflammatory disorders [Gurung, 2015]. Counteracting these mitochondrial impairments with HAELR/GZ and maintaining mitochondrial homeostasis could inturn reduce excess inflammatory response, the hallmark pathology of pancreatitis.

5.4.9 Histopathological studies

Figure 5.13 represents the photomicrographs of pancreas from all the experimental rats during the study of pancreato-protective effect of HAELR.

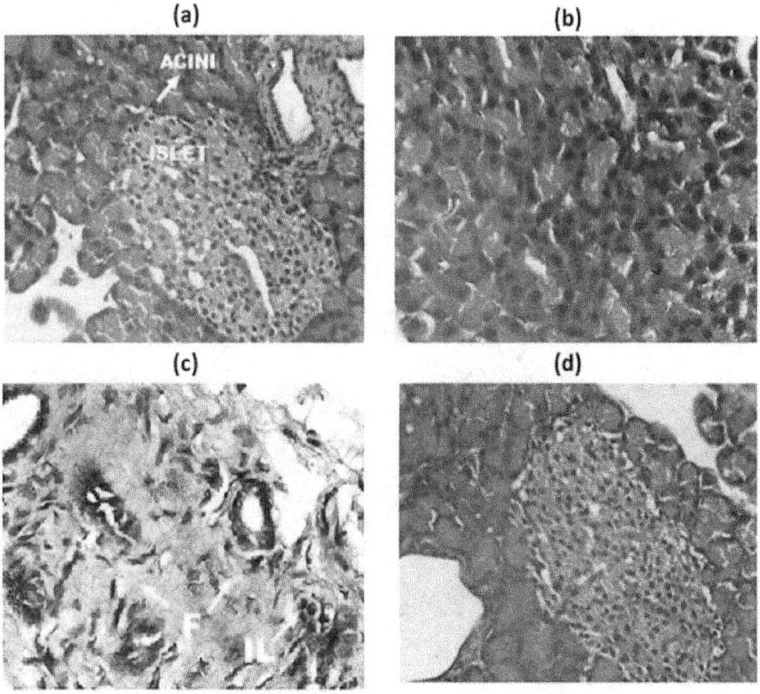

Figure 5.13 Pancreato-protective effect of hydroalcoholic licorice root extract evidenced by histological observation

Photomicrograph (H&E stained,400X magnification) of pancreas (a) Control group, showing normal tissue architecture with intact acini and islets; (b)HAELR control, without any abnormal pathological changes; (c)EtOH + Cer induced pancreatitis group, showing inflammatory cell infiltration (IL) and fibrosis (F); (d)HAELR co-administered group, with restored tissue architecture.

Pancreatic sections from control and HAELR control showed normal tissue architecture with acini and islets, without any abnormal pathological changes (Figure 5.13a and Figure 5.13b).

Sections of the pancreas from pancreatitis-induced rats, showed neutrophil infiltration and fibrotic changes (Figure 5.13c). Tissue architecture of pancreas of HAELR coadministered (100 mg/kg) group was shown with improved and less significant pathological changes (Figure 5.13d).

Figure 5.14 represents the photomicrographs of pancreas from all the experimental rats during the study of pancreato-protective effect of GZ.

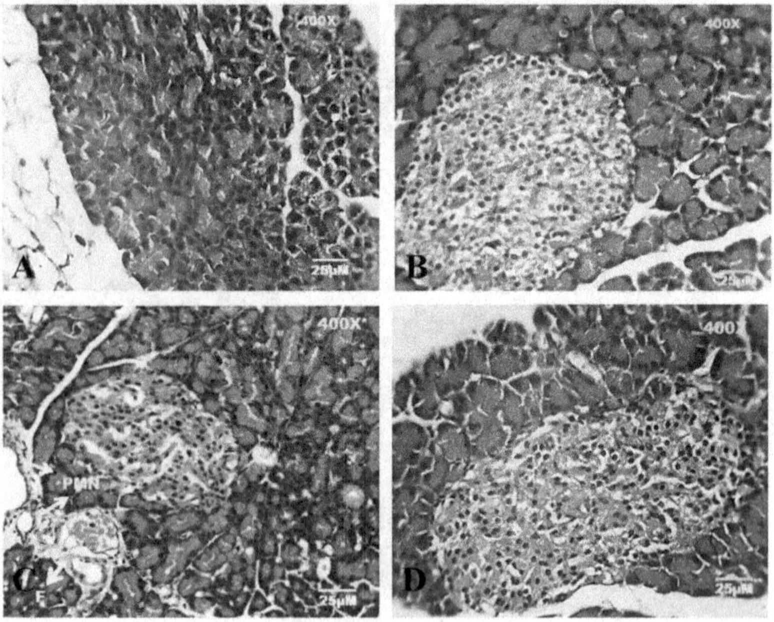

Figure 5.14 Pancreato-protective effect of Glycyrrhizin evidenced by histological observation

Photomicrograph (H&E stained,400X magnification) of pancreas (A)Control group, showing normal tissue architecture; (B)GZ control, without any abnormal pathological changes; (C)EtOH + Cer induced pancreatitis group, revealing polymorphonuclear infiltration (PMN) and fibrosis (F); (D)GZ co-administered group, with near-normal tissue architecture.

Pancreatic sections from control and GZ control showed normal tissue architecture (Figure 5.14A and Figure 5.14B). Histological observations in the study evidenced a prominent neutrophil infiltration and mild fibrosis in pancreatic sections of pancreatitis-induced rats (Figure 5.14C) which is a characteristic feature of CP. This was found to be counteracted by GZ, as observed in pancreatic sections of GZ coadministered rats (Figure 5.14D). The reason behind this excessive inflammatory response in pancreatitis rats is perhaps the NF-κB activation, as noted from RT-PCR study.

5.5 Molecular docking analysis

GZ is subjected to *in silico* molecular docking study to further acknowledge its pancreatoprotectivity. Molecular docking was conducted between GZ and the UPR component proteins like GRP78 and ATF4. The visualized hydrogen bond interactions between GZ and GRP78, GZ and ATF4 using Acceryls Discovery Studio Visualizer were shown in **figure 5.15** and **figure 5.16**, respectively.

Two hydrogen bond interactions were found between GZ and GRP78 at residues LYS81, THR85 with the docking energy of -5.82 kcal/mol as shown in **table 5.25**. Two hydrogen bond interactions were found between GZ and ATF4 at residues LYS315, LYS316 with the docking energy of -5.8 kcal/mol as shown in **table 5.26**. A good binding affinity was observed in the molecular docking study, between GZ and GRP78, GZ and ATF4.

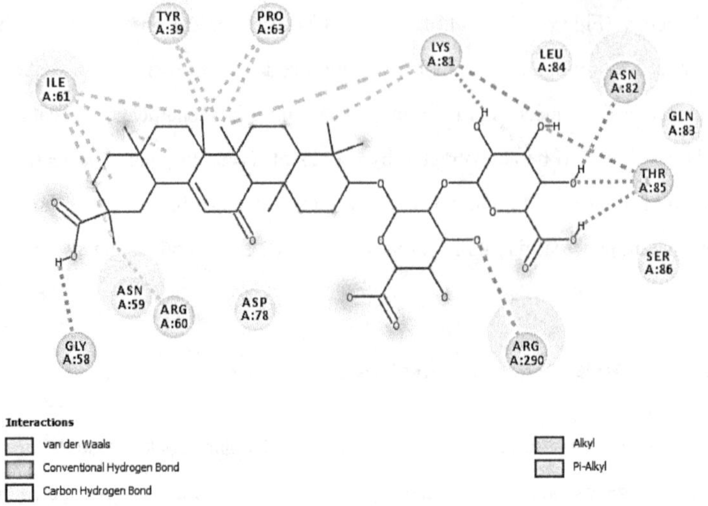

Table 5.25 Molecular docking studies of Glycyrrhizin with GRP78

GRP78		Glycyrrhizin	Distance (Å)	Binding Energy (Kcal/mol)
Residue	Atom			
GLY58	O	H	2.46	-5.82
THR85	N	O	2.97	
THR85	N	O	2.80	
THR85	OG1	O	2.56	
THR85	OG1	O	2.72	
THR85	OG1	H	2.01	
ASN82	O	H	2.33	
LYS81	O	H	2.02	
ARG290	NH1	O	2.95	

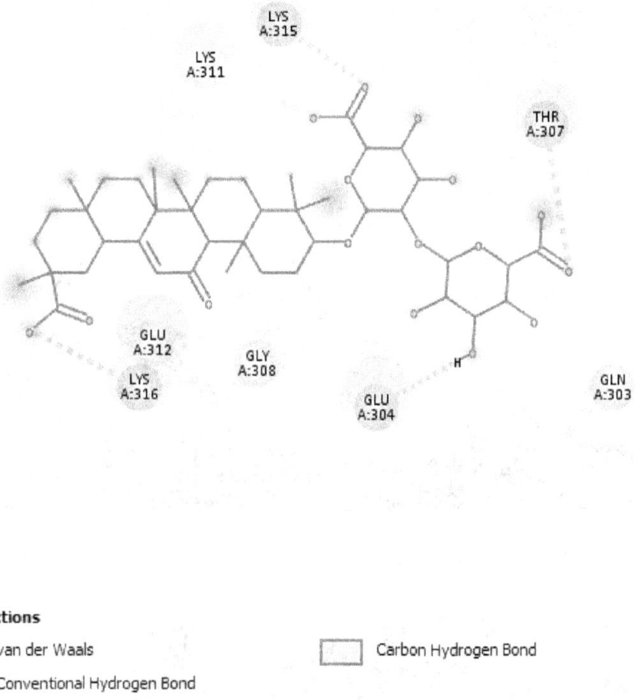

Table 5.26 Molecular docking studies of Glycyrrhizin with ATF4

ATF4		Glycyrrhizin	Distance (Å)	Binding Energy (Kcal/mol)
Residue	Atom			
LYS316	NZ	O	3.18	-5.82
LYS316	NZ	O	2.64	
LYS315	NZ	O	2.84	
GLU304	OE1	H	2.33	
THR307	OG1	O	2.81	

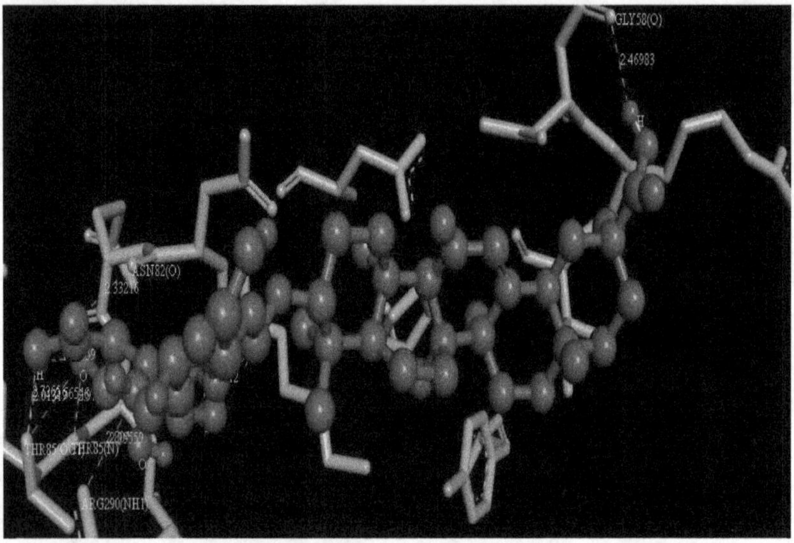

Figure 5.15 Molecular docking studies of Glycyrrhizin with GRP78

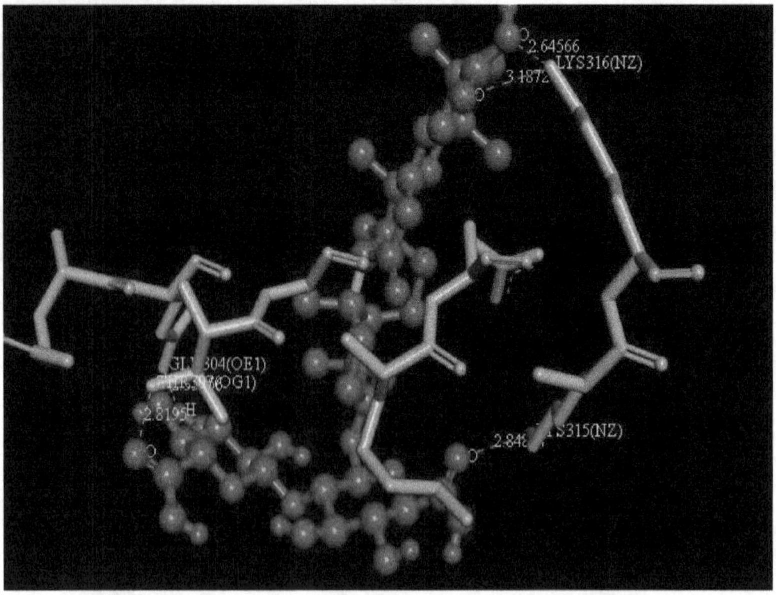

Figure 5.16 Molecular docking studies of Glycyrrhizin with ATF4

From the docking study it is clear that, GZ was found to bind to GRP78 suppressing GRP78s induction, thereby inhibiting ER stress and ultimately ameliorating CP. Many previous studies have shown, decrease in the expression of GRP78, markedly reduce necrosis and attenuate the severity of inflammation in pancreatic acinar cells [Liu Y,2014]. Similarly, compounds like quercetin aglycone (Quer) and its glycosylated derivative, quercetin 3-*O*-xyloside (Quer-Xyl) were reported to be effective against pancreatitis by regulating GRP78 [Seo JY, 2019].

Upregulated ATF4 signaling acts mostly through CHOP, a transcription factor that directs ER stress-induced cytokine production and inflammation in response to ER stress. CHOP mediates the secretion of cytokine IL-1 β [Nishitoh H,2012]. GZ was found to bind to ATF4 suppressing ATF4 induction and may be its downstream targets like CHOP. Pro-inflammatory mechanisms of the CHOP-mediated pathway may also occur through NF-κB activation. A similar study indicated that melatonin, an anti-inflammatory molecule prevents the severity of experimental pancreatitis by acting on these ER stress markers [Zhao Q,2018].

The present in silico docking study demonstrated that ER stress pathway, which was activated in CP and served an important role in exacerbating pancreatic injury, NF-κB activation and the expression of pro-inflammatory cytokines is attenuated by GZ. Since glycyrrhizin shows a good binding affinity towards GRP78 and ATF4, it could hold a great promise for use in the treatment of CP in future after thorough clinical study. **Table 5.27** represents molecular properties of GZ described through docking analysis. During drug discovery, the drug-likeness and rule of 5 proposed by Lipinski predicts that, poor absorption is more likely to happen when there are more than 5 H-bond donors (8 in GZ), 10 H-bond acceptors (13 in GZ), the molecular weight is greater than 500 (822.942 in GZ), the calculated Log P is greater than 5 (2.2456 in GZ) and number of rotatable bonds exceed 15 (7 in GZ). However, it is very unfavorable for GZ to follow Lipinski's rule of five as it is characterized by three violations.

Table 5.27 Molecular properties of Glycyrrhizin

Descriptor	Value
Molecular weight	822.942
Log P	2.2456
#Rotatable Bonds	7
# Hydrogen bond acceptors	13
#Hydrogen bond donors	8
Surface Area	337.426

However, Lipinski specifically mentions that the Rule of 5 of drugability, only holds for compounds that are not substrates for active transporters [Lipinski C,2001]. Even added the fact that, most of the leads obtained through high-throughput screening tends to have higher molecular weights. The fact that, GZ belongs to "beyond Rule-of-5" is throwing light to investigate the presence of uptake transporters for GZ. A huge fraction of the Ro5 violators are generally found to be natural products or their derivatives [Benet LZ,2016]. Macrolide antibiotics (clarithromycin, erythromycin and roxithromycin), immunosuppressants (cyclosporine, sirolimus, tacrolimus and everolimus), HIV protease inhibitors (atazanavir, lopinavir, nelfinavir and tipranavir) and tyrosine kinase inhibitors (lapatinib and nilotinib) etc are the other drugs observed to show higher violation numbers, but still are good drugs of choice for various ailments. So, realistic assessment of compounds is necessitated to know their actual suitability during test drug research.

A drug that falls outside of the Rule of 5 and is orally available is assumed to be a substrate for a transporter. It has been documented previously that, after oral administration, GZ gets slowly absorbed from the gut and converted by the colonic microflora into the deglycosylated metabolite glycyrrhetic acid, which can be absorbed easily [Yu K,2012]. Existence of GZ transporters like Oatp1b2 in rats, OATP1B (OATP1B1 and OATP1B3) in humans were reported independently. These transporters facilitate hepatobiliary excretion of GZ by mediating the compound's uptake from blood besides assisting the circulation of GZ [Dong J,2018]. All these facts propose GZ as a good therapeutic drug for pancreatitis, and can be considered for further drug development.

6. SUMMARY

Chronic pancreatitis arises when the pancreas becomes injured by long-standing inflammation, mostly caused by alcohol abuse. Inflammation impairs pancreatic functions gradually with long-standing abdominal pain as the major clinical symptom. Poor functional pancreas causes improper digestion of fats, altered blood sugar levels, nutritional deficiencies and weight loss. If left unmonitored, CP can increase the risk of pancreatic cancer. Diagnosis is challenging in CP as symptoms are similar to that of ulcers, gallstones, irritable bowel syndrome, or even pancreatic cancer. Blood tests, which can detect the digestive enzyme leakage, out of the pancreas into the bloodstream, when the pancreas is inflamed are very reliable markers.

Traditional herbal medicine, which take advantage of the plant extracts, is dominating the treatment of chronic diseases in recent times. Here by, we focused one such traditional herb, *Glycyrrhiza glabra* and its major phytoconstituent glycyrrhizin against alcohol and cerulein-induced rat model of CP. The present study was aimed to give scientific evidence for the pancreato-protective effect of HAELR and GZ which are traditionally used for inflammation related disorders. Experimental rats were subjected to alcohol and cerulein induced inflammation and treated with the test drugs. HAELR and glycyrrhizin exhibited excellent pancreato-protective activity against various pathobiologies of CP and, the obtained results are summarized below:

- HAELR was subjected to GCMS analysis, and it revealed the presence of biologically important phytochemicals like 3-hydroxy-3,4,5,7-tetramethoxyflavone, jaceidin triacetate and undecane.

- HPLC-UV analysis conducted, revealed the presence of flavonoids like rutin, luteolin, thymoquinone and galangin at a concentration of 0.9 mg/g, 0.6 mg/g, 0.5 mg/g, and 1.3 mg/g, respectively and saponins like glycyrrhzin at a concentration of 0.02 mg/g in HAELR.

- The predicted oral rat LD_{50} for GZ was estimated by nearest neighbor method using TEST software tool. It was found to be 88.39 mg/kg body weight.

- The LD_{50} value of HAELR was found to be greater than 5000 mg/kg body weight.

- Acute toxicity study was carried out with the concentrations of 500, 1000, 2000, 4000 and 5000 mg/kg b.wt. of HAELR for 14days and sub-chronic toxicity study with concentrations of 50, 100, 200,400 and 500 mg/kg b.wt. for 90 days. No adverse effects were noted. No mortality was observed upto 5000mg/kg b. wt, highlighting the safety of HAELR. This was evidenced by biochemical, hematological and histopathological investigations besides various other general observations.

- There observed no notable changes in morphology, behavior or physiology during acute and chronic exposures of HAELR.And there observed no significant changes either in the body weight or relative organ weights.

- Acute and chronic exposures of HAELR did not cause any prominent alteration in the liver,heart and kidney functions as indicated by their respective biochemical markers. No drastic change was observed either in the oxidative status or hematological system, upon acute and chronic exposures of HAELR.

- The histopathological examinations were conducted on liver, kidney, heart, pancreas and brain tissues. Acute and chronic exposures of HAELR did not cause any abnormalities or tissue architecture alterations.

- Dose response studies were conducted with 25, 50, 100 and 200 mg/kg b.wt. of HAELR and 2.5, 5, 10 and 20 mg/kg b.wt. of GZ. The pancreatic markers like lipase and amylase, and inflammatory markers like MPO, caspase-1, IL-1 β and IL-18 were assessed. Both the markers were found elevated during EtOH and Cer-induced pancreatitis. HAELR/GZ co-administrations were observed to restore them. The doses of 100 mg/kg b.wt of HAELR and 10 mg/kg b.wt of

GZ, which exhibited maximum pancreato-protective effect against EtOH and Cer-induced pancreatitis, were selected for carrying out further investigations.

- The therapeutic efficacy of HAELR and GZ against EtOH and Cer-induced pancreatitis was investigated in detail and the results are: The pancreatitis marker enzymes like lipase and amylase activities were found elevated in serum significantly, upon administration of EtOH and Cer. HAELR/GZ co-administrations observed to have restored these levels significantly confirming their protectivity against pancreatic injury.

- Cellular oxidative stress was measured through total peroxide content, TAC and OSI; GSH, GPx, SOD and CAT activities. Lipid peroxidation was measured through determinations of TBARS and 4-HNE.Oxidative stress and lipid peroxidation were found elevated significantly during EtOH and Cer-induced pancreatitis. Whereas, HAELR/GZ co-administration found to ameliorate these pathological changes.

- Inflammation was measured through activity of pancreatic MPO, and serum levels of caspase-1, IL-1 β, and IL-18. It was found increased significantly during EtOH and Cer-induced pancreatitis. The levels of these inflammatory mediators were found restored with HAELR/GZ co-administrations indicating the attenuation of pancreatic inflammation by HAELR and GZ.

- mRNA expression of NF-κB was studied to monitor inflammation in pancreas. It was found elevated significantly during EtOH and Cer-induced pancreatitis, as evidenced from RT-PCR analysis. It was observed to be ameliorated with HAELR/GZ co-administrations.

- mRNA expression of the UPR genes (ATF4, GRP78, CHOP and XBP1) were studied to monitor ER stress in pancreas. They were found upregulated significantly indicating the chronically activated ER stress during EtOH and Cer-induced pancreatitis. HAELR/GZ co-administrations were observed to ameliorate the increased expression, underlining their role in protecting against pathologic ER stress in CP.

- Oxidative stress was assessed in pancreatic mitochondria. A significant decrease in GSH content, antioxidant enzymes (GPx, SOD, CAT) and a significant increase in lipid peroxidation products (TBARS,4-HNE) were observed in mitochondria during EtOH and Cer-induced pancreatitis, indicating association of CP with mitochondrial oxidative stress. HAELR/GZ co-administrations were recorded to enhance the anti-oxidative capacity of mitochondria as evidenced from the attenuated levels of antioxidants.

- The intra-mitochondrial free calcium levels were determined and were found increased significantly upon EtOH and Cer administration. This is due to the gradual release of Ca 2+ from ER under the influence of alcoholic metabolites like FAEEs. This increase was not observed with HAELR/GZ co-administrations emphasizing attenuation of [Ca 2+] m overload in mitochondria by HAELR/GZ.

- Mitochondrial functional alteration was monitored through complex-1 activity. Pronounced inhibition of complex-1 activity of mitochondrial respiratory chain was observed during EtOH and Cer-induced pancreatitis, pointing out the decline in energy formation. It was observed to be re-established upon HAELR/GZ co-administrations.

- Histopathological studies were conducted to add more evidence for the therapeutic efficacy of HAELR and GZ. It revealed the presence of prominent inflammation and fibrosis during EtOH and Cer-induced pancreatitis. These pathological alterations in pancreatic tissue architecture were found to be minimized by HAELR/GZ co-administration.

- The Spearman's rank correlation test was conducted between GRP78 vs 4-HNE; CHOP vs IL-1β, $[Ca^{2+}]_m$; $[Ca^{2+}]_m$ vs complex-1, TBARS and GSH; CHOP vs NF-κB. In this study, a correlated effect was observed between ER stress and mitochondrial dysfunction, the key mechanisms contributing to the pathobiology of CP as indicated by a positive correlation found between GRP78 vs 4-HNE and CHOP vs IL-1β, $[Ca^{2+}]_m$.

- An *insilico* molecular docking analysis was carried out to understand the effect of GZ on ER stress. The docking energy between GZ vs GRP78 and ATF4 was found to be -5.82 kcal/mol and -5.8 kcal/mol respectively. This analysis gives base level evidence for the binding affinity between GZ and the target proteins GRP78 and ATF4.This would be true and mimic, the affinity and interaction invivo.

7. CONCLUSION

Results of the current investigation has shown that, HAELR is rich in phytochemicals with a wide variety of pharmacological activities. HAELR/ glycyrrhizin plays a key role in decreasing the pathological modifications of alcohol and cerulein-induced pancreatitis. HAELR/glycyrrhizin exerts significant pancreato-protective properties, probably by mitigating the ER stress and its consequent mitochondrial dysfunction and oxidative stress, and there by the inflammation. In this regard, HAELR/GZ inhibits ER stress by downregulating its UPR components- ATF4, GRP78, CHOP and XBP1. Furthermore, HAELR/glycyrrhizin downregulates expression of NF-κB and its consequent maturation of pro-inflammatory cytokines, responsible for regulating the level of inflammation in pancreas. GZ was observed to have had a good binding affinity towards GRP78 and ATF4 in *insilico* molecular docking. Thus, HAELR/GZ can be considered as potent drugs for the treatment of pancreatitis which targets ER stress followed by mitochondrial dysfunction and NF-κB activation, resulting in the mitigation of maturation and release of pro-inflammatory cytokines in pancreas, offering protection to the organ.

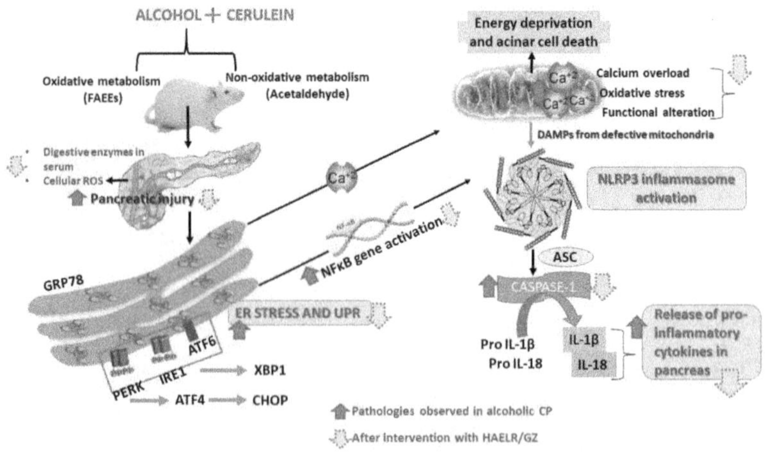

The tentative highlight on the mode of action of HAELR/GZ

8. FUTURE PROSPECTS OF THESTUDY

The study warrants the need to extrapolate the obtained results of this animal study, to clinical trials and check whether this kind of intervention with HAELR/GZ could reduce the disease severity of alcoholic CP in human beings also.

9. BIBLIOGRAPHY

Abed A, Minaiyan M, Ghannadi A, Mahzouni P, Babavalian MR. Effect of Echium amoenum Fisch. et Mey a traditional Iranian herbal remedy in an experimental model of acute pancreatitis. International Scholarly Research Notices. 2012;2012.

Aebi H. Catalase in vitro. InMethods in enzymology 1984 Jan 1;105: 121-126.

Aghdassi AA, Mayerle J, Christochowitz S, Weiss FU, Sendler M, Lerch MM. Animal models for investigating chronic pancreatitis. Fibrogenesis & tissue repair. 2011 Dec;4(1):1-6.

Ahmadi A, Nikkhoo B, Mokarizadeh A, Rahmani MR, Fakhari S, Mohammadi M, Jalili A. An optimised mouse model of chronic pancreatitis with a combination of ethanol and cerulein. Central-European journal of immunology. 2016;41(1):54.

Aljancić I, Stanković M, Tešević V, Vujisić L, Vajs V, Milosavljević S. Protective effect on human lymphocytes of some flavonoids isolated from two Achillea species. Natural product communications. 2010 May;5(5):19.

Allen SL. Regulatory aspects of acute neurotoxicity assessment: In, Hayes' Handbook of Pesticide Toxicology. Edn 3, Elsevier, Chicago, USA, 2010, 587-602.

Al-Rubaye AF, Hameed IH, Kadhim MJ. A review: uses of gas chromatography-mass spectrometry (GC-MS) technique for analysis of bioactive natural compounds of some plants. International Journal of Toxicological and Pharmacological Research. 2017 Mar;9(1):81-5.

American Botanical Council https://www.herbalgram.org/resources/herbmedpro/herb-list/glycyrrhiza-glabra-g-uralensis/

Apte MV, Haber PS, Norton ID, Wilson JS. Alcohol and the pancreas. Addict Biol, 1998;3(2):137-50.

Apte MV, Pirola RC, Wilson JS. Alcohol and the pancreas. Pancreapedia: The Exocrine Pancreas Knowledge Base; 2016. Doi: 10.3998/panc.2016.17

Apte MV, Pirola RC, Wilson JS. Mechanisms of alcoholic pancreatitis. Journal of gastroenterology and hepatology. 2010 Dec;25(12):1816-26.

Apte MV, Wilson JS. Stellate cell activation in alcoholic pancreatitis. Pancreas. 2003 Nov 1;27(4):316-20.

Archer-Lahlou E, Escrieut C, Clerc P, et al. Molecular mechanism underlying partial and full agonism mediated by the human cholecystokinin-1 receptor. J Biol Chem 2005;280:10664-10674.

Arnould M, Tassa A, Ferrand A, et al. The G-protein-coupled CCK2 receptor associates with phospholipase Cgamma1.FEBS Lett 2004;568:89-93.

Atkinson MA, Campbell-Thompson M, Kusmartseva I, Kaestner KH. Organisation of the human pancreas in health and in diabetes. Diabetologia. 2020 Oct;63(10):1966-73.

Baba M, Shigeta S. Antiviral activity of glycyrrhizin against varicella-zoster virus in vitro. Antiviral research. 1987 Feb 1;7(2):99-107.

Bae GS, Park KC, Koo BS, Choi SB, Jo IJ, Choi CM, Song HJ, Park SJ. The inhibitory effects of Nardostachys jatamansi on alcoholic chronic pancreatitis. BMB reports. 2012;45(7):402-7.

Bailly C, Vergoten G. Glycyrrhizin: An alternative drug for the treatment of COVID-19 infection and the associated respiratory syndrome?. Pharmacology & Therapeutics. 2020 Jun 24:107618.

Balakrishnan V, Unnikrishnan AG, Thomas V, Choudhuri G, Veeraraju P, Singh SP, Garg P, Pai CG, Devi RN, Bhasin D, Jayanthi V. Chronic pancreatitis. A prospective nationwide study of 1,086 subjects from India. JOP: Journal of the pancreas. 2008 Sep 2;9(5):593-600.

Bariweni MW, Yibala OI, Ozolua RI. Toxicological studies on the aqueous leaf extract of Pavetta crassipes (K. Schum) in rodents. Journal of Pharmacy & Pharmacognosy Research. 2018 Jan 1;6(1):1-6.

Batandier C, Leverve X, Fontaine E. Opening of the mitochondrial permeability transition pore induces reactive oxygen species production at the level of the respiratory chain complex I. Journal of Biological Chemistry. 2004 Apr 23;279(17):17197-204.

Batiha GE, Beshbishy AM, El-Mleeh A, Abdel-Daim MM, Devkota HP. Traditional uses, bioactive chemical constituents, and pharmacological and toxicological activities of Glycyrrhiza glabra L.(Fabaceae). Biomolecules. 2020 Mar;10(3).

Bedoya LM, Beltrán M, García-Pérez J, Obregón-Calderón P, Callies O, Jímenez IA, Bazzocchi IL, Alcamí J. Promiscuous, multi-target lupane-type triterpenoids inhibits wild type and drug resistant HIV-1 replication through the interference with several targets. Frontiers in pharmacology. 2018 Apr 18;9:358.

Benet LZ, Hosey CM, Ursu O, Oprea TI. BDDCS, the rule of 5 and drugability. Advanced drug delivery reviews. 2016 Jun 1;101:89-98.

Bhardwaj P, Yadav RK. Chronic pancreatitis: role of oxidative stress and antioxidants. Free radical research. 2013 Nov 1;47(11):941-9.

Bhattacharjee A, Shashidhara SC, Saha S. Evaluation of acute and sub-chronic oral toxicity study of ethanolic extract of Crataeva nurvala Buch-ham stem bark on experimental Wistar rats. Group. 2013; 14:5.

Bhattamisra SK, Siang TC, Rong CY, Annan NC, Sean EH, Xi LW, Lyn OS, Shan LH, Choudhury H, Pandey M, Gorain B. Type-3c diabetes mellitus, diabetes of exocrine pancreas-an update. Current diabetes reviews. 2019 Oct 1;15(5):382-94.

Bhosale VV, Banerjee D. Scientific Validation of Herbal Medicine. InHerbal Medicine in India. Springer, Singapore, 2020, 573-579.

Biczo G, Vegh ET, Shalbueva N, Mareninova OA, Elperin J, Lotshaw E, Gretler S, Lugea A, Malla SR, Dawson D, Ruchala P. Mitochondrial dysfunction, through impaired autophagy, leads to endoplasmic reticulum stress, deregulated lipid metabolism, and pancreatitis in animal models. Gastroenterology. 2018 Feb 1;154(3):689-703.

Biswas SK. Does the interdependence between oxidative stress and inflammation explain the antioxidant paradox?. Oxidative medicine and cellular longevity. 2016 Oct;2016.

Boaru SG, Borkham-Kamphorst E, Van de Leur E, Lehnen E, Liedtke C, Weiskirchen R. NLRP3 inflammasome expression is driven by NF-κB in cultured hepatocytes. Biochemical and biophysical research communications. 2015 Mar 13;458(3):700-6.

Booth DM, Murphy JA, Mukherjee R, Awais M, Neoptolemos JP, Gerasimenko OV, Tepikin AV, Petersen OH, Sutton R, Criddle DN. Reactive oxygen species induced by bile acid induce apoptosis and protect against necrosis in pancreatic acinar cells. Gastroenterology. 2011 Jun 1;140(7):2116-25.

Bouhlel A, Mosbah IB, Abdallah NH, Ribault C, Viel R, Mannaï S, Corlu A, Abdennebi HB. Thymoquinone prevents endoplasmic reticulum stress and mitochondria-induced apoptosis in a rat model of partial hepatic warm ischemia reperfusion. Biomedicine & Pharmacotherapy. 2017 Oct 1;94:964-73.

Bouhrim M, Ouassou H, Choukri M, Mekhfi H, Ziyyat A, Legssyer A, Aziz M, Bnouham M. Hepatoprotective effect of Opuntia dillenii seed oil on CCl4 induced acute liver damage in rat. Asian Pacific Journal of Tropical Biomedicine. 2018;8(5):254.

Bowers GN, McComb RB. Measurement of total alkaline phosphatase activity in human. Clinical Chemistry. 1975; 21(13):1988-1995.

Boxhoorn L, Voermans RP, van Santvoort HC, Besselink MG. Acute pancreatitis–Authors' reply. The Lancet. 2021 Jan 23;397(10271):280.

Bradford MM. A rapid and sensitive method for the quantitation of microgram quantities of protein utilizing the principle of protein-dye binding. Analytical Biochemistry. 1976; 72(1-2): 248-254.

Bradley PP, Christensen RD, Rothstein G. Cellular and extracellular myeloperoxidase in pyogenic inflammation. Blood. 1982; 60 (3): 618-622.

Bravo R, Gutierrez T, Paredes F, Gatica D, Rodriguez AE, Pedrozo Z, Chiong M, Parra V, Quest AF, Rothermel BA, Lavandero S. Endoplasmic reticulum: ER stress regulates mitochondrial bioenergetics. The international journal of biochemistry & cell biology. 2012 Jan 1;44(1):16-20.

Brookes PS, Yoon Y, Robotham JL, Anders MW, Sheu SS. Calcium, ATP, and ROS: a mitochondrial love-hate triangle. Am J Physiol Cell Physiol, 2004; 287(4): C817-33.

Brough D, Le Feuvre RA, Wheeler RD, Solovyova N, Hilfiker S, Rothwell NJ, Verkhratsky A. Ca2+ stores and Ca2+ entry differentially contribute to the release of IL-1β and IL-1α from murine macrophages. The Journal of Immunology. 2003 Mar 15;170(6):3029-36.

Cao SS, Kaufman RJ. Endoplasmic reticulum stress and oxidative stress in cell fate decision and human disease. Antioxid Redox Signal, 2014;21(3):396-413.

Chaudhari N, Talwar P, Parimisetty A, Lefebvre d'Hellencourt C, Ravanan P. A molecular web: endoplasmic reticulum stress, inflammation, and oxidative stress. Front Cell Neurosci, 2014;8: 213.

Cho JA, Park E. Curcumin utilizes the anti-inflammatory response pathway to protect the intestine against bacterial invasion. Nutrition research and practice. 2015 Apr;9(2):117.

Choi JW, Jeong JH, Jo IJ, Kim DG, Shin JY, Kim MJ, Choi BM, Shin YK, Song HJ, Bae GS, Park SJ. Preventive Effects of Gardenia jasminoides on cerulein-induced chronic pancreatitis. The American Journal of Chinese Medicine. 2020 May 20;48(04):987-1003.

Christian AG, Kechi EL, Oshie NC, John AD, Nwakaego EM, Ahunna AG, Nwobodo NN. Haematological and biochemical changes after exposure to Maerua crassifolia ethanol leaf extract in rats. Journal of Applied Pharmaceutical Science. 2017;7(6):136-140.

Clemens DL, Wells MA, Schneider KJ, Singh S. Molecular mechanisms of alcohol associated pancreatitis. World J Gastrointest Pathophysiol, 2014;5(3):147.

Collins LV, Hajizadeh S, Holme E, Jonsson IM, Tarkowski A. Endogenously oxidized mitochondrial DNA induces in vivo and in vitro inflammatory responses. Journal of leukocyte biology. 2004 Jun;75(6):995-1000.

Conwell DL, Lee LS, Yadav D, Longnecker DS, Miller FH, Mortele KJ, Levy MJ, Kwon R, Lieb JG, Stevens T, Toskes PP. American Pancreatic Association Practice Guidelines in Chronic Pancreatitis: evidence-based report on diagnostic guidelines. Pancreas. 2014 Nov;43(8):1143.

Cooley MM, Jones EK, Gorelick FS, Groblewski GE. Pancreatic Acinar Cell Protein Synthesis, Intracellular Transport, and Export. Pancreapedia: The Exocrine Pancreas Knowledge Base. 2020 Dec 21.

Courreges AP, Najenson AC, Vatta MS, Bianciotti LG. Atrial natriuretic peptide attenuates endoplasmic reticulum stress in experimental acute pancreatitis. Biochimica et Biophysica Acta (BBA)-Molecular Basis of Disease. 2019 Feb 1;1865(2):485-93.

Criddle DN, Gerasimenko JV, Baumgartner HK, Jaffar M, Voronina S, Sutton R, Petersen OH, Gerasimenko OV. Calcium signalling and pancreatic cell death: apoptosis or necrosis? Cell Death Differ, 2007;14(7):1285-94.

Criddle DN, Murphy J, Fistetto G, Barrow S, Tepikin AV, Neoptolemos JP, Sutton R, Petersen OH. Fatty acid ethyl esters cause pancreatic calcium toxicity via inositol trisphosphate receptors and loss of ATP synthesis. Gastroenterology. 2006 Mar 1;130(3):781-93.

Damle M. Glycyrrhiza glabra (Liquorice)-a potent medicinal herb. International Journal of Herbal Medicine. 2014;2(2):132-6.

De Boeck K. Cystic fibrosis in the year 2020: A disease with a new face. Acta Paediatrica. 2020 May;109(5):893-9.

Delierneux C, Kouba S, Shanmughapriya S, Potier-Cartereau M, Trebak M, Hempel N. Mitochondrial calcium regulation of redox signaling in cancer. Cells. 2020 Feb;9(2):432.

Deng X, Wang L, Elm MS, Gabazadeh D, Diorio GJ, Eagon PK, Whitcomb DC. Chronic alcohol consumption accelerates fibrosis in response to cerulein-induced pancreatitis in rats. The American journal of pathology. 2005 Jan 1;166(1):93-106.

Detaille D, Pasdois P, Sémont A, Dos Santos P, Diolez P. An old medicine as a new drug to prevent mitochondrial complex I from producing oxygen radicals. PloS one. 2019 May 2;14(5):e0216385.

Dhananjayan K. Molecular docking study characterization of rare flavonoids at the Nac-binding site of the first bromodomain of BRD4 (BRD4 BD1). Journal of Cancer Research. 2015 Mar 22;2015.

Dinarello CA, Ikejima T, Warner SJ, Orencole SF, Lonnemann G, Cannon JG, Libby P. Interleukin 1 induces interleukin 1. I. Induction of circulating interleukin 1 in rabbits in vivo and in human mononuclear cells in vitro. The Journal of Immunology. 1987 Sep 15;139(6):1902-10.

Dong J, Olaleye OE, Jiang R, Li J, Lu C, Du F, Xu F, Yang J, Wang F, Jia W, Li C. Glycyrrhizin has a high likelihood to be a victim of drug–drug interactions mediated by hepatic organic anion- transporting polypeptide 1B1/1B3. British journal of pharmacology. 2018 Sep;175(17):3486-503.

Draper HH, Hadley M. Malondialdehyde determination as index of lipid peroxidation. Methods Enzymol. 1990; 186:421-431.

Duggan SN, Chonchubhair HM, Lawal O, O'Connor DB, Conlon KC. Chronic pancreatitis: A diagnostic dilemma. World journal of gastroenterology. 2016 Feb 21;22(7):2304.

Ejeh SA, Abalaka SE, Usende IL, Alimi YA, Oyelowo FO. Acute toxicity, oxidative stress response and clinicopathological changes in Wistar rats exposed to aqueous extract of Uvaria chamae leaves. Scientific African. 2019 May 1;3:e00068.

Endo M, Mori M, Akira S, Gotoh T. C/EBP Homologous Protein (CHOP) Is Crucial for the Induction of Caspase-11 and the Pathogenesis of Lipopolysaccharide-Induced Inflammation. The Journal of Immunology. 2006 May 15;176(10): 6245-53.

Erhirhie EO, Ihekwereme CP, Ilodigwe EE. Advances in acute toxicity testing: strengths, weaknesses and regulatory acceptance. Interdisciplinary toxicology. 2018;11(1):5-12.

Etemad B, Whitcomb DC. Chronic pancreatitis: diagnosis, classification, and new genetic developments. Gastroenterology. 2001 Feb 1;120(3):682-707.

Fakhari S, Abdolmohammadi K, Panahi Y, Nikkhoo B, Peirmohammadi H, Rahmani MR, Moghadam AS, Jalili A. Glycyrrhizin attenuates tissue injury and reduces neutrophil accumulation in experimental acute pancreatitis. International journal of clinical and experimental pathology. 2014;7(1):101.

Feissner RF, Skalska J, Gaum WE, Sheu SS. Crosstalk signaling between mitochondrial Ca2+ and ROS. Frontiers in bioscience: a journal and virtual library. 2009 Jan 1;14:1197.

Flohé L, Günzler WA. Methods in Enzymology 1984; 105 (1): 114-121.

Folch E, Gelpi E, Rosello-Catafau J, Closa D. Free radicals generated by xanthine oxidase mediate pancreatitis-associated organ failure. Digestive diseases and sciences. 1998 Nov;43(11):2405-10.

Frulloni L, Patrizi F, Bernardoni L, Cavallini G. Pancreatic hyperenzymemia: clinical significance and diagnostic approach. Jop, 2005; 6(6):536-51.

Fuchs TC, Hewitt P. Biomarkers for drug-induced renal damage and nephrotoxicity-an overview for applied toxicology. Journal of the American Association of Pharmaceutical Scientists. 2011; 13(4):615-631.

Fürst R, Zündorf I. Plant-derived anti-inflammatory compounds: hopes and disappointments regarding the translation of preclinical knowledge into clinical progress. Mediators of inflammation. 2014 Oct;2014.

Gaman L, Dragos D, Vlad A, Robu GC, Radoi MP, Stroica L, Badea M, Gilca M. Phytoceuticals in acute pancreatitis: targeting the balance between apoptosis and necrosis. Evidence-Based Complementary and Alternative Medicine. 2018 Jan 1;2018.

Gardner TB, Adler DG, Forsmark CE, Sauer BG, Taylor JR, Whitcomb DC. ACG clinical guideline: chronic pancreatitis. Official journal of the American College of Gastroenterology| ACG. 2020 Mar 1;115(3):322-39.

Gibo J, Ito T, Kawabe K, Hisano T, Inoue M, Fujimori N, Oono T, Arita Y, Nawata H. Camostat mesilate attenuates pancreatic fibrosis via inhibition of monocytes and pancreatic stellate cells activity. Laboratory investigation. 2005 Jan;85(1):75-89.

Ginwala R, Bhavsar R, Chigbu DG, Jain P, Khan ZK. Potential role of flavonoids in treating chronic inflammatory diseases with a special focus on the anti-inflammatory activity of apigenin. Antioxidants. 2019 Feb;8(2):35.

Godkar PB, Godkar DP. Textbook of medical laboratory technology. Bhalani; 2003.

Gomaa AA, Abdel-Wadood YA. The potential of glycyrrhizin and licorice extract in combating COVID-19 and associated conditions. Phytomedicine Plus. 2021 Feb 17:100043.

González-Reyes S, Santillán-Cigales JJ, Jiménez-Osorio AS, Pedraza-Chaverri J, Guevara-Guzmán R. Glycyrrhizin ameliorates oxidative stress and inflammation in hippocampus and olfactory bulb in lithium/pilocarpine-induced status epilepticus in rats. Epilepsy research. 2016 Oct 1;126:126-33.

Grijalba MT, Vercesi AE, Schreier S. Ca2+-induced increased lipid packing and domain formation in submitochondrial particles. A possible early step in the mechanism of Ca2+-stimulated generation of reactive oxygen species by the respiratory chain. Biochemistry. 1999 Oct 5;38(40):13279-87.

Grynkiewicz G, Poenie M, Tsien RY. A new generation of Ca2+ indicators with greatly improved fluorescence properties. Journal of biological chemistry. 1985 Mar 25;260(6):3440-50.

Gukovskaya AS, Gukovsky I, Algül H, Habtezion A. Autophagy, inflammation, and immune dysfunction in the pathogenesis of pancreatitis. Gastroenterology. 2017 Nov 1;153(5):1212-26.

Gukovskaya AS, Hosseini S, Satoh A, Cheng JH, Nam KJ, Gukovsky I, Pandol SJ. Ethanol differentially regulates NF-κB activation in pancreatic acinar cells through calcium and protein kinase C pathways. American Journal of Physiology-Gastrointestinal and Liver Physiology. 2004 Feb;286(2):G204-13.

Gukovsky I, Gukovskaya AS, Blinman TA, Zaninovic V, Pandol SJ. Early NF-κB activation is associated with hormone-induced pancreatitis. American Journal of Physiology-Gastrointestinal and Liver Physiology. 1998 Dec 1;275(6): G1402-14.

Gukovsky I, Lugea A, Shahsahebi M, Cheng JH, Hong PP, Jung YJ, Deng QG, French BA, Lungo W, French SW, Tsukamoto H. A rat model reproducing key pathological responses of alcoholic chronic pancreatitis. American Journal of Physiology-Gastrointestinal and Liver Physiology. 2008 Jan;294(1): G68-79.

Guo R, Ma H, Gao F, Zhong L, Ren J. Metallothionein alleviates oxidative stress-induced endoplasmic reticulum stress and myocardial dysfunction. Journal of molecular and cellular cardiology. 2009 Aug 1;47(2):228-37.

Gurung P, Lukens JR, Kanneganti TD. Mitochondria: diversity in the regulation of the NLRP3 inflammasome. Trends Mol Med, 2015;21(3):193-201.

Haber PS, Wilson JS, Apte MV, Pirola RC. Fatty acid ethyl esters increase rat pancreatic lysosomal fragility. The Journal of laboratory and clinical medicine. 1993 Jun 1;121(6):759-64.

Han R, Wang Y, Dabbous M, Liang S, Qiu T, Toumi M. Chinese clinical studies for pharmacological treatments of coronavirus disease 2019 (COVID-19).2020

Handa SS. An overview of extraction techniques for medicinal and aromatic plants. Extraction technologies for medicinal and aromatic plants. 2008;1.

Hassan HS, Sule MI, Musa AM, Musa KY, Abubakar MS, Hassan AS. Anti-inflammatory activity of crude saponin extracts from five Nigerian medicinal plants. African Journal of Traditional, Complementary and Alternative Medicines. 2012;9(2):250-5.

Hayes AW, Loomis TA. Loomis's essentials of toxicology. Elsevier, 1996.

Hegyi P, Párniczky A, Lerch MM, Sheel AR, Rebours V, Forsmark CE, Del Chiaro M, Rosendahl J, de-Madaria E, Szücs Á, Takaori K. International consensus guidelines for risk factors in chronic pancreatitis. Recommendations from the working group for the international consensus guidelines for chronic pancreatitis in collaboration with the international association of pancreatology, the American pancreatic association, the Japan pancreas society, and European pancreatic club. Pancreatology. 2020 Apr 8.

Hong YP, Deng WH, Guo WY, Shi Q, Zhao L, You YD, Mei FC, Zhou Y, Wang CY, Chen C, Yu J. Inhibition of endoplasmic reticulum stress by 4-phenylbutyric acid prevents vital organ injury in rat acute pancreatitis. American Journal of Physiology-Gastrointestinal and Liver Physiology. 2018 Nov 1;315(5):G838-47.

Hoque R, Mehal WZ. Inflammasomes in pancreatic physiology and disease. Am J Physiol Gastrointest Liver Physiol 2015; 308(8): G643-651.

Hotta Y, Ishikawa N, Ohashi N, Matsui K. Effects of SM-20550, a selective Na+-H+ exchange inhibitor, on the ion transport of myocardial mitochondria. Molecular and cellular biochemistry. 2001 Mar;219(1):83-90.

https://www.epa.gov/chemical-research/toxicity-estimation-software-tool-test#methodologies

Hu P, Han Z, Couvillon AD, Kaufman RJ, Exton JH. Autocrine tumor necrosis factor alpha links endoplasmic reticulum stress to the membrane death receptor pathway through IRE1α-mediated NF-κB activation and down-regulation of TRAF2 expression. Molecular and cellular biology. 2006 Apr 15;26(8):3071-84.

Huan CC, Wang HX, Sheng XX, Wang R, Wang X, Mao X. Glycyrrhizin inhibits porcine epidemic diarrhea virus infection and attenuates the proinflammatory responses by inhibition of high mobility group box-1 protein. Archives of virology. 2017 Jun;162(6):1467-76.

Huang D, Qi DF. Damarane sapogenins from ginseng, their uses as anti-cancer agents. US Patent 6888014B2. 2005.

Huang H, Liu Y, Daniluk J, Gaiser S, Chu J, Wang H, Li ZS, Logsdon CD, Ji B. Activation of nuclear factor-κB in acinar cells increases the severity of pancreatitis in mice. Gastroenterology, 2013; 144(1):202-10.

Huang W, Cash N, Wen L, Szatmary P, Mukherjee R, Armstrong J, Chvanov M, Tepikin AV, Murphy MP, Sutton R, Criddle DN. Effects of the mitochondria-targeted antioxidant mitoquinone in murine acute pancreatitis. Mediators of Inflammation. 2015 Jan 1;2015.

Irving HM, Samokhvalov AV, Rehm J. Alcohol as a risk factor for pancreatitis. A systematic review and meta-analysis. Jop. 2009 Jul 6;10(4):387.

JainD. Chronic pancreatitis. PathologyOutlines.com website. https://www.pathology outlines.com/topic/pancreaschronic.html. Accessed March 17th, 2021.

Janiak A, Leśniowski B, Jasińska A, Pietruczuk M, Małecka-Panas E. Interleukin 18 as an early marker or prognostic factor in acute pancreatitis. Przeglad gastroenterologiczny. 2015;10(4):203.

Javed MA, Wen L, Awais M, Latawiec D, Huang W, Chvanov M, Schaller S, Bordet T, Michaud M, Pruss R, Tepikin A. TRO40303 Ameliorates Alcohol-Induced Pancreatitis Through Reduction of Fatty Acid Ethyl Ester–Induced Mitochondrial Injury and Necrotic Cell Death. Pancreas. 2018 Jan;47(1):18.

Jekabsone A, Ivanoviene L, Brown GC, Borutaite V. Nitric oxide and calcium together inactivate mitochondrial complex I and induce cytochrome c release. Journal of molecular and cellular cardiology. 2003 Jul 1;35(7):803-9.

Joint FA, WHO Expert Committee on Food Additives, World Health Organization. Evaluation of certain food additives: sixty-third report of the Joint FAO. World Health Organization; 2005.

Kaja S, Payne AJ, Naumchuk Y, Koulen P. Quantification of lactate dehydrogenase for cell viability testing using cell lines and primary cultured astrocytes. Current protocols in toxicology. 2017; 72(1): 2-6.

Kakkar P, Das B, Viswanathan PN. A modified spectrophotometric assay of superoxide dismutase (1984). Indian J. Biochem. Biophys. 1984; 21:130-132.

Kamei J, Nakamura R, Ichiki H, Kubo M. Antitussive principles of *Glycyrrhiza radix*, a main component of Kampo preparations Bakumondo-to (Mai-men-dongtang).E J Pharm 2003; 69:159-163.

Kang R, Lotze MT, Zeh HJ, Billiar TR, Tang D. Cell death and DAMPs in acute pancreatitis. Molecular medicine. 2014 Jan;20(1):466-77.

Keller J, Layer P. Diagnosis of pancreatic exocrine insufficiency in chronic pancreatitis. Pancreapedia: The Exocrine Pancreas Knowledge Base. 2015 Sep 14.

Khan AA, Alsahli MA, Rahmani AH. Myeloperoxidase as an active disease biomarker: recent biochemical and pathological perspectives. Medical sciences. 2018 Jun;6(2):33.

Kikuta K, Masamune A, Satoh M, Suzuki N, Shimosegawa T. 4-hydroxy-2, 3-nonenal activates activator protein-1 and mitogen-activated protein kinases in rat pancreatic stellate cells. World J Gastroenterol 2004; 10(16): 2344.

Kim H. Cerulein pancreatitis: Oxidative stress, inflammation, and apoptosis. Gut Liver 2008; 2(2): 74.

Kim JH, Kismali G, Gupta SC. Natural products for the prevention and treatment of chronic inflammatory diseases: Integrating traditional medicine into modern chronic diseases care. 2018.

Kim SW, Jin Y, Shin JH, Kim ID, Lee HK, Park S, Han PL, Lee JK. Glycyrrhizic acid affords robust neuroprotection in the postischemic brain via anti-inflammatory effect by inhibiting HMGB1 phosphorylation and secretion. Neurobiology of disease. 2012 Apr 1;46(1):147-56.

King J. The dehydrogenases or oxidoreductases — Lactate dehydrogenase. Practical Clinical Enzymology.1965 (b); 83–93.

King J. The transferases — alanine and aspartate transaminases. Practical Clinical Enzymology.1965 (a); 121–138.

Kinter M, Grimminger LC, Gillies PJ, Shimshick EJ, Ayers C. Whole Blood and Plasma Concentrations of 4-Hydroxy-2-nonenal in Watanabe Heritable Hyperlipidemic Versus New Zealand White Rabbits. Biochemical and Biophysical Research Communications. 1994; 199(2): 671-675.

Kirk GR, White JS, McKie L, Stevenson M, Young I, Clements WB, Rowlands BJ. Combined antioxidant therapy reduces pain and improves quality of life in chronic pancreatitis. Journal of gastrointestinal surgery. 2006 Apr;10(4):499-503.

Klochkov A, Kudaravalli P, Sun Y. Alcoholic Pancreatitis. StatPearls [Internet]. 2020 Jan 23.

Korpela T, Udd M, Mustonen H, Ristimäki A, Haglund C, Seppänen H, Kylänpää L. Association between chronic pancreatitis and pancreatic cancer: A 10- year retrospective study of endoscopically treated and surgical patients. International journal of cancer. 2020 Sep 1;147(5):1450-60.

Kregiel D, Berlowska J, Witonska I, Antolak H, Proestos C, Babic M, Babic L, Zhang B. Saponin-based, biological-active surfactants from plants. Application and characterization of surfactants. 2017 Jul 5;6(1):184-205.

Kubisch CH, Gukovsky I, Lugea A, Pandol SJ, Kuick R, Misek DE, Hanash SM, Logsdon CD. Long-term ethanol consumption alters pancreatic gene expression in rats: a possible connection to pancreatic injury. Pancreas. 2006 Jul 1;33(1):68-76.

Kubisch CH, Logsdon CD. Secretagogues differentially activate endoplasmic reticulum stress responses in pancreatic acinar cells. American Journal of Physiology-Gastrointestinal and Liver Physiology. 2007 Jun;292(6):G1804-12.

Kussmaul L, Hirst J. The mechanism of superoxide production by NADH: ubiquinone oxidoreductase (complex I) from bovine heart mitochondria. Proceedings of the National Academy of Sciences. 2006 May 16;103(20):7607-12.

Kwiecien S, Jasnos K, Magierowski M, Sliwowski Z, Pajdo R, Brzozowski B, et al. Lipid peroxidation, reactive oxygen species and antioxidative factors in the pathogenesis of gastric mucosal lesions and mechanism of protection against oxidative stress-induced gastric injury. J Physiol Pharmacol 2014; 65(5): 613-622.

Kwon YJ, Son DH, Chung TH, Lee YJ. A review of the pharmacological efficacy and safety of licorice root from corroborative clinical trial findings. Journal of medicinal food. 2020 Jan 1;23(1):12-20.

Langer D, Czarczynska-Goslinska B, Goslinski T. Glycyrrhetinic acid and its derivatives in infectious diseases. Current Issues in Pharmacy and Medical Sciences. 2016 Sep 1;29(3):118-23.

LaRusch J, Whitcomb DC. Genetics of pancreatitis. Current opinion in gastroenterology. 2011 Sep;27(5):467.

Lawrence T. The nuclear factor NF-κB pathway in inflammation. Cold Spring Harbor perspectives in biology. 2009 Dec 1;1(6):a001651.

Lee SK, Choi JW, Kim MJ, Kim DG, Shin JY, Zhou Z, Jo IJ, Song HJ, Bae GS, Park SJ. Piperine ameliorates the severity of fibrosis via inhibition of TGF-β/SMAD signaling in a mouse model of chronic pancreatitis. Molecular medicine reports. 2019 Oct 1;20(4):3709-18.

Li J, Xia X, Ke Y, Nie H, Smith MA, Zhu X. Trichosanthin induced apoptosis in HL-60 cells via mitochondrial and endoplasmic reticulum stress signaling pathways. Biochimica et Biophysica Acta (BBA)-General Subjects. 2007 Aug 1;1770(8):1169-80.

Li JY, Cao HY, Liu P, Cheng GH, Sun MY. Glycyrrhizic acid in the treatment of liver diseases: literature review. Biomed Res Int, 2014;2014:872139.

Li X, Sun R, Liu R. Natural products in licorice for the therapy of liver diseases: Progress and future opportunities. Pharmacological research. 2019 Jun 1; 144:210-26.

Li YL, Guo H, Zhao YQ, Li AF, Ren YQ, Zhang JW. Quercetin protects neuronal cells from oxidative stress and cognitive degradation induced by amyloid β-peptide treatment. Molecular medicine reports. 2017 Aug 1;16(2):1573-7.

Limonta P, Moretti RM, Marzagalli M, Fontana F, Raimondi M, Montagnani Marelli M. Role of endoplasmic reticulum stress in the anticancer activity of natural compounds. International journal of molecular sciences. 2019 Jan;20(4):961.

Lipinski C. a, Lombardo, F., Dominy, BW & Feeney, PJ Experimental and computational approaches to estimate solubility and permeability in drug discovery and development settings. Adv. Drug Deliv. Rev. 2001;46(1-3):3.

Lipinski CA. Lead-and drug-like compounds: the rule-of-five revolution. Drug Discovery Today: Technologies. 2004 Dec 1;1(4):337-41.

Liu Y, Yang L, Chen KL, Zhou B, Yan H, Zhou ZG, Li Y. Knockdown of GRP78 promotes apoptosis in pancreatic acinar cells and attenuates the severity of cerulein and LPS induced pancreatic inflammation. PLoS One. 2014 Mar 18;9(3):e92389.

Logsdon CD, Ji B. The role of protein synthesis and digestive enzymes in acinar cell injury. Nature reviews Gastroenterology & hepatology. 2013 Jun;10(6):362.

Lugea A, Gukovsky I, Gukovskaya AS, Pandol SJ. Nonoxidative ethanol metabolites alter extracellular matrix protein content in rat pancreas. Gastroenterology. 2003 Dec 1;125(6):1845-59.

Lugea A, Tischler D, Nguyen J, Gong J, Gukovsky I, French SW, Gorelick FS, Pandol SJ. Adaptive unfolded protein response attenuates alcohol-induced pancreatic damage. Gastroenterology. 2011 Mar 1;140(3):987-97.

Lugea A, Waldron RT, Pandol SJ. Pancreatic adaptive responses in alcohol abuse: Role of the unfolded protein response. Pancreatology, 2015;15(4): S1-5.

Majumdar AP, Vesenka GD, Dubick MA, Yu GS, DeMorrow JM, Geokas MC. Morphological and biochemical changes of the pancreas in rats treated with acetaldehyde. American Journal of Physiology-Gastrointestinal and Liver Physiology. 1986 May 1;250(5):G598-606.

Majumder S, Chari ST. Chronic pancreatitis. The Lancet. 2016 May 7;387(10031): 1957-66.

Maksoud HA, Magid AD, Mostafa YM, Elharrif MG, Sorour RI, Sorour MI. Ameliorative effect of liquorice extract versus silymarin in experimentally induced chronic hepatitis: A biochemical and genetical study. Clinical Nutrition Experimental. 2019 Feb 1;23:69-79.

Manzo-Avalos S, Saavedra-Molina A. Cellular and mitochondrial effects of alcohol consumption. Int J Environ Res Public Health, 2010;7(12):4281-304.

Marchi S, Patergnani S, Pinton P. The endoplasmic reticulum–mitochondria connection: one touch, multiple functions. Biochim Biophys Acta, 2014 ;1837(4):461-9.

Marrache F, Tu SP, Bhagat G, Pendyala S, Österreicher CH, Gordon S, et al. Overexpression of interleukin-1β in the murine pancreas results in chronic pancreatitis. Gastroenterology 2008; 135(4): 1277-1287.

Martin T. User's Guide for TEST (Toxicity Estimation Software Tool)-A Program to Estimate Toxicity from Molecular Structure, 2016.

Martinon F, Mayor A, Tschopp J. The inflammasomes: guardians of the body. Annual review of immunology. 2009 Apr 23;27:229-65.

Martucciello S, Masullo M, Cerulli A, Piacente S. Natural products targeting ER stress, and the functional link to mitochondria. International journal of molecular sciences. 2020 Jan;21(6):1905.

Masamune A, Watanabe T, Kikuta K, Satoh K, Shimosegawa T. NADPH oxidase plays a crucial role in the activation of pancreatic stellate cells. American Journal of Physiology-Gastrointestinal and Liver Physiology. 2008 Jan;294(1):G99-108.

McGill MR. The past and present of serum aminotransferases and the future of liver injury biomarkers. Experimental and Clinical Sciences Journal. 2016; 15: 817.

Meng Y, Ma QY, Kou XP, Xu J. Effect of resveratrol on activation of nuclear factor kappa-B and inflammatory factors in rat model of acute pancreatitis. World journal of gastroenterology: WJG. 2005 Jan 28;11(4):525.

Midha S, Khajuria R, Shastri S, Kabra M, Garg PK. Idiopathic chronic pancreatitis in India: phenotypic characterisation and strong genetic susceptibility due to SPINK1 and CFTR gene mutations. Gut. 2010 Jun 1;59(6):800-7.

Miller NJ, Rice-Evans C, Davies MJ, Gopinathan V, Milner A. A novel method for measuring antioxidant capacity and its application to monitoring the antioxidant status in premature neonates. Clinical science. 1993 Apr 1;84(4): 407-12.

Min M, Patel B, Han S, Bocelli L, Kheder J, Vaze A, Wassef W. Exocrine pancreatic insufficiency and malnutrition in chronic pancreatitis: identification, treatment, and consequences. Pancreas. 2018 Sep;47(8):1015.

Miyazawa T. Determination of phospholipid hydroperoxides in human blood plasma by a chemiluminescence-HPLC assay. Free Radical Biology and Medicine. 1989 Jan 1;7(2):209-18.

Molla MD, Akalu Y, Geto Z, Dagnew B, Ayelign B, Shibabaw T. Role of Caspase-1 in the Pathogenesis of Inflammatory-Associated Chronic Noncommunicable Diseases. Journal of Inflammation Research. 2020;13:749.

Moron MS, De Pierre JW, Vik BM. Levels of glutathione, glutathione reductase and glutathione - S - transferase activities in rat, lung and liver. Biochem. Biophys. Acta. 1979; 582: 3170-3185.

Mukherjee M, Bhaskaran N, Srinath R, Shivaprasad HN, Allan JJ, Shekhar D, Agarwal A. Anti-ulcer and antioxidant activity of GutGard TM.Indian journal of experimental biology.2010;48:269-274.

Muratov EN, Bajorath J, Sheridan RP, Tetko IV, Filimonov D, Poroikov V, Oprea TI, Baskin II, Varnek A, Roitberg A, Isayev O. QSAR without borders. Chemical Society Reviews. 2020 Jun 8;49(11):3525-64.

Nadkarni KM. [Indian materia medica]; Dr. KM Nadkarni's Indian materia medica: with Ayurvedic, Unani-Tibbi, Siddha, allopathic, homeopathic, naturopathic & home remedies, appendices & indexes. 1. Popular Prakashan; 1996.

Natelson, S, Scott, ML, Beffa, C. Rapid methods for estimation of urea in biologic fluids; by means of reaction between diacetyl and urea. American Journal of Clinical Pathology. 1951; 21: 275–281.

Ning JW, Zhang Y, Yu MS, Gu ML, Xu J, Usman A, et al. Emodin alleviates intestinal mucosal injury in rats with severe acute pancreatitis via the caspase-1 inhibition. Hepatobiliary Pancreat Dis Int 2017; 16(4): 431-436.

Nirogi R, Goyal VK, Jana S, Pandey SK, Gothi A. What suits best for organ weight analysis: review of relationship between organ weight and body/brain weight for rodent toxicity studies. International Journal of Pharmaceutical Sciences and Research. 2014;5(4):1525-1532.

Nishitoh H. CHOP is a multifunctional transcription factor in the ER stress response. J Biochem, 2012;151(3):217-9.

Nitsche C, Maertin S, Scheiber J, Ritter CA, Lerch MM, Mayerle J. Drug-induced pancreatitis. Current gastroenterology reports. 2012 Apr;14(2):131-8.

Norton ID, Apte MV, Haber PS, McCaughan GW, Pirola RC, Wilson JS. Cytochrome P4502E1 is present in rat pancreas and is induced by chronic ethanol administration. Gut. 1998 Mar 1;42(3):426-30.

Obafemi TF, Yu P, Li J, Davis JM, Liu K, Cheng B, Zhao X, Shen Q, Younes M, Ko TC, Cao Y. Comparable Responses in Male and Female Mice to Cerulein-Induced Chronic Pancreatic Injury and Recovery. JOP: Journal of the pancreas. 2018 Sep;19(5):236.

Odinokova IV, Sung KF, Mareninova OA, Hermann K, Evtodienko Y, Andreyev A, Gukovsky I, Gukovskaya AS. Mechanisms regulating cytochrome c release in pancreatic mitochondria. Gut, 2009;58(3):431-42.

Olayode OA, Daniyan MO, Olayiwola G. Biochemical, hematological and histopathological evaluation of the toxicity potential of the leaf extract of Stachytarpheta cayennensis in rats. Journal of Traditional and Complementary Medicine. 2019.

Olesen SS, Krarup H, Poulsen JL, Christensen JH, Sheel AR, Sutton R, Greenhalf W, Halloran C, Drewes AM. Pancreas-specific plasma amylase for assessment and diagnosis of chronic pancreatitis: New insights on an old topic. United European gastroenterology journal. 2019 Aug;7(7):955-64.

Omar HR, Komarova I, El-Ghonemi M, Fathy A, Rashad R, Abdelmalak HD, Yerramadha MR, Ali Y, Helal E, Camporesi EM. Licorice abuse: time to send a warning message. Therapeutic advances in endocrinology and metabolism. 2012 Aug;3(4):125-38.

Organisation for Economic Co-operation and Development. Test No. 423: Acute oral Toxicity-Acute toxic class method. OECD Publishing, 2002.

Osei- Bimpong A, McLean R, Bhonda E, Lewis SM. The use of the white cell count and haemoglobin in combination as an effective screen to predict the normality of the full blood count. International journal of laboratory hematology. 2012 Feb;34(1):91-7.

Otsuki M, Yamamoto M, Yamaguchi T. Animal models of chronic pancreatitis. Gastroenterology research and practice. 2010 Dec 14;2010.

Pahl HL, Baeuerle PA. Activation of NF- κB by ER stress requires both Ca2+ and reactive oxygen intermediates as messengers. FEBS letters. 1996 Aug 26;392(2):129-36.

Pal R, Cristan EA, Schnittker K, Narayan M. Rescue of ER oxidoreductase function through polyphenolic phytochemical intervention: implications for subcellular traffic and neurodegenerative disorders. Biochemical and Biophysical Research Communications. 2010 Feb 19;392(4):567-71.

Pan YL. The effects of glycyrrhizin on acute pancreatitis in mice. Eur Rev Med Pharmacol Sci. 2014 Jan 1;18(24):3943-7.

Panahi Y, Fakhari S, Mohammadi M, Rahmani MR, Hakhamaneshi MS, Jalili A. Glycyrrhizin down-regulates CCL2 and CXCL2 expression in cerulein-stimulated pancreatic acinar cells. American journal of clinical and experimental immunology. 2015;4(1):1.

Pandol SJ, Periskic S, Gukovsky I, Zaninovic V, Jung Y, Zong Y, Solomon TE, Gukovskaya AS, Tsukamoto H. Ethanol diet increases the sensitivity of rats to pancreatitis induced by cholecystokinin octapeptide. Gastroenterology. 1999 Sep 1;117(3):706-16.

Pastorino G, Cornara L, Soares S, Rodrigues F, Oliveira MB. Liquorice (Glycyrrhiza glabra): A phytochemical and pharmacological review. Phytotherapy research. 2018 Dec;32(12):2323-39.

Perbtani Y, Forsmark CE. Update on the diagnosis and management of exocrine pancreatic insufficiency. F1000Research. 2019;8.

Pereira CA, Carlos D, Ferreira NS, Silva JF, Zanotto CZ, Zamboni DS, Garcia VD, Ventura DF, Silva JS, Tostes RC. Mitochondrial DNA promotes NLRP3 inflammasome activation and contributes to endothelial dysfunction and inflammation in type 1 diabetes. Frontiers in physiology. 2020 Jan 17;10: 1557.

Ploeger B, Mensinga T, Sips A, Seinen W, Meulenbelt J, DeJongh J. The pharmacokinetics of glycyrrhizic acid evaluated by physiologically based pharmacokinetic modeling. Drug metabolism reviews. 2001 Jan 1;33(2):125-47.

PradyotBikashKar Mahapatra, Joydip Tripathi , Rishi Vashishth. Clinical study of chronic pancreatitis (tikshnoshna pitta) treated with some ayurvedic medicaments. International Ayurvedic Medical Journal.2017;5 (2)

Ralla T, Salminen H, Braun K, Edelmann M, Dawid C, Hofmann T, Weiss J. Investigations into the Structure-Function Relationship of the Naturally-Derived Surfactant Glycyrrhizin: Emulsion Stability. Food Biophysics. 2020 Jan 18:1-9.

Ramsey ML, Conwell DL, Hart PA. Complications of chronic pancreatitis. Digestive diseases and sciences. 2017 Jul 1;62(7):1745-50.

Raveendra KR, Srinivasa V, Sushma KR, Allan JJ, Goudar KS, Shivaprasad HN, Venkateshwarlu K, Geetharani P, Sushma G, Agarwal A. An extract of Glycyrrhiza glabra (GutGard) alleviates symptoms of functional dyspepsia: a randomized, double-blind, placebo-controlled study. Evidence-Based Complementary and Alternative Medicine. 2012 Jan 1;2012.

Rawla P, Sunkara T, Gaduputi V. Epidemiology of pancreatic cancer: global trends, etiology and risk factors. World journal of oncology. 2019 Feb;10(1):10.

Reed A, Gorelick F. Animal models of chronic pancreatitis. Pancreapedia: The Exocrine Pancreas Knowledge Base. 2014 Oct 2.

Ren Z, Wang X, Xu M, Yang F, Frank JA, Ke ZJ, Luo J. Binge ethanol exposure causes endoplasmic reticulum stress, oxidative stress and tissue injury in the pancreas. Oncotarget. 2016 Aug 23;7(34):54303.

Rizzuto R, Pinton P, Carrington W, Fay FS, Fogarty KE, Lifshitz LM, Tuft RA, Pozzan T. Close contacts with the endoplasmic reticulum as determinants of mitochondrial Ca2+ responses. Science. 1998 Jun 12;280(5370):1763-6.

Robles L, Vaziri ND, Ichii H. Role of oxidative stress in the pathogenesis of pancreatitis: effect of antioxidant therapy. Pancreatic disorders & therapy. 2013 Apr 1;3(1):112.

Sah RP, Garg SK, Dixit AK, Dudeja V, Dawra RK, Saluja AK. Endoplasmic reticulum stress is chronically activated in chronic pancreatitis. Journal of Biological Chemistry. 2014 Oct 3;289(40):27551-61.

Saha S, Gouda TS, Srinivas SV. Preliminary Phytochemical Analysis and Oral Acute Toxicity Study of the Leaves of Baccaurea ramiflora and Microcos paniculata. Saudi Journal of Medical and Pharmaceutical Sciences. 2017;3(6):444-9.

Salim S, Kalam MA, Yusuf A, Khanday S, Shafi S, Mohammad I. Asl-us-Sus (Glycyrrhiza glabra L.), a great munzij-i-balgham (concotive of phlegm) drug of Unani system of medicine: a review. Int J Unani Integ Med. 2018;2(3):16-9.

Sandoval DI, Gukovskaya AN, Reavey PA, Gukovsky SO, Sisk AB, Braquet PI, Pandol SJ, Poucell-Hatton SI. The role of neutrophils and platelet-activating factor in mediating experimental pancreatitis. Gastroenterology. 1996 Oct 1;111(4):1081-91.

Sankaran SJ, Xiao AY, Wu LM, Windsor JA, Forsmark CE, Petrov MS. Frequency of progression from acute to chronic pancreatitis and risk factors: a meta-analysis. Gastroenterology. 2015 Nov 1;149(6):1490-500.

Schneider A, Haas SL, Hildenbrand R, Siegmund S, Reinhard I, Nakovics H, et al. Enhanced expression of interleukin-18 in serum and pancreas of patients with chronic pancreatitis. World J Gastroenterol 2006; 12(40): 6507.

Schroder K, Tschopp J. The inflammasomes. cell. 2010 Mar 19;140(6):821-32.

Sen S, Chakraborty R. Revival, modernization and integration of Indian traditional herbal medicine in clinical practice: Importance, challenges and future. Journal of traditional and complementary medicine. 2017 Apr 1;7(2):234-44.

Seo JY, Pandey RP, Lee J, Sohng JK, Namkung W, Park YI. Quercetin 3-O-xyloside ameliorates acute pancreatitis in vitro via the reduction of ER stress and enhancement of apoptosis. Phytomedicine. 2019 Mar 1;55:40-9.

Seyhun E, Malo A, Schäfer C, Moskaluk CA, Hoffmann RT, Göke B, Kubisch CH. Tauroursodeoxycholic acid reduces endoplasmic reticulum stress, acinar cell damage, and systemic inflammation in acute pancreatitis. American Journal of Physiology-Gastrointestinal and Liver Physiology. 2011 Nov;301(5):G773-82.

Shalbueva N, Mareninova OA, Gerloff A, Yuan J, Waldron RT, Pandol SJ, Gukovskaya AS. Effects of oxidative alcohol metabolism on the mitochondrial permeability transition pore and necrosis in a mouse model of alcoholic pancreatitis. Gastroenterology. 2013 Feb 1;144(2):437-46.

Shapiro H, Singer P, Halpern Z, Bruck R. Polyphenols in the treatment of inflammatory bowel disease and acute pancreatitis. Gut. 2007 Mar 1;56(3): 426-36.

Shen A, Kim HJ, Oh GS, Lee SB, Lee SH, Pandit A, Khadka D, Choe SK, Kwak SC, Yang SH, Cho EY. NAD+ augmentation ameliorates acute pancreatitis through regulation of inflammasome signalling. Scientific reports. 2017 Jun 7;7(1):1-3.

Shenbagam M, Nalini N. Dose response effect of rutin a dietary antioxidant on alcohol- induced prooxidant and antioxidant imbalance–a histopathologic study. Fundamental & clinical pharmacology. 2011;25(4):493-502.

Sheu SS, Sharma VK. A novel technique for quantitative measurement of free Ca2+ concentration in rat heart mitochondria. J Physiol, 1999;518(2):577-84.

Shimada K, Crother TR, Karlin J, Chen S, Chiba N, Ramanujan VK, Vergnes L, Ojcius DM, Arditi M. Caspase-1 dependent IL-1β secretion is critical for host defense in a mouse model of Chlamydia pneumoniae lung infection. PloS one. 2011 Jun 23;6(6):e21477.

Simsek O, Kocael A, Kocael P, Orhan A, Cengiz M, Balcı H, et al. Inflammatory mediators in the diagnosis and treatment of acute pancreatitis: Pentraxin-3, procalcitonin and myeloperoxidase. Arch Med Sci 2018; 14(2): 288.

Slot C. Plasma creatinine determination a new and specific Jaffe reaction method. Scandinavian Journal Of Clinical And Laboratory Investigation. 1965; 17(4):381-387.

Sostres C, Gargallo CJ, Arroyo MT, Lanas A. Adverse effects of non-steroidal anti-inflammatory drugs (NSAIDs, aspirin and coxibs) on upper gastrointestinal tract. Best practice & research Clinical gastroenterology. 2010 Apr 1;24(2): 121-32.

St-Pierre J, Buckingham JA, Roebuck SJ, Brand MD. Topology of superoxide production from different sites in the mitochondrial electron transport chain. Journal of Biological Chemistry. 2002 Nov 22;277(47):44784-90.

Strowig T, Henao-Mejia J, Elinav E, Flavell R. Inflammasomes in health and disease. nature. 2012 Jan;481(7381):278-86.

Sun Q, Zhong W, Zhang W, Zhou Z. Defect of mitochondrial respiratory chain is a mechanism of ROS overproduction in a rat model of alcoholic liver disease: role of zinc deficiency. Am J Physiol Gastrointest Liver Physiol, 2016; 310(3): G205-14.

Suyama K, Ohmuraya M, Hirota M, Ozaki N, Ida S, Endo M, Araki K, Gotoh T, Baba H, Yamamura KI. C/EBP homologous protein is crucial for the acceleration of experimental pancreatitis. Biochemical and biophysical research communications. 2008 Feb 29;367(1):176-82.

Tam AB, Mercado EL, Hoffmann A, Niwa M. ER stress activates NF-κB by integrating functions of basal IKK activity, IRE1 and PERK. PloS one. 2012 Oct 26;7(10):e45078.

Telek G, Regöly-Mérei J, Kovács GC, Simon L, Nagy Z, Hamar J, Jakab F. The first histological demonstration of pancreatic oxidative stress in human acute pancreatitis. Hepato-gastroenterology. 2001 Sep 1;48(41):1252-8.

Teo S, Stirling D, Thomas S, Hoberman A, Kiorpes A, Khetani V. A 90-day oral gavage toxicity study of d-methylphenidate and d, l-methylphenidate in Sprague–Dawley rats. Toxicology. 2002 Oct 15;179(3):183-96.

Thakkar S, Anklam E, Xu A, Ulberth F, Li J, Li B, Hugas M, Sarma N, Crerar S, Swift S, Hakamatsuka T. Regulatory landscape of dietary supplements and herbal medicines from a global perspective. Regulatory Toxicology and Pharmacology. 2020 Jul 1;114:104647.

Thirumal Y, Laavu S. HPLC profile of medicinal plant extracts and its application in aquaculture. J Aquacult Res Dev. 2017;8(484):2-6.

Toskes PP, Dawson W, Curington C, Levy NS, Fitzgerald C. Non-diabetic retinal abnormalities in chronic pancreatitis. New England Journal of Medicine. 1979 Apr 26;300(17):942-6.

Trenker M, Fertschai I, Malli R, Graier WF. UCP2/3—likely to be fundamental for mitochondrial Ca 2+ uniport. Nat Cell Biol, 2008; 10(11):1237–40.

Tretter L, Adam-Vizi V. Generation of reactive oxygen species in the reaction catalyzed by α-ketoglutarate dehydrogenase. Journal of Neuroscience. 2004 Sep 8;24(36):7771-8.

Trumbeckaite S, Kuliaviene I, Deduchovas O, Kincius M, Baniene R, Virketyte S, Bukauskas D, Jansen E, Kupčinskas L, Borutaite V, Gulbinas A. Experimental acute pancreatitis induces mitochondrial dysfunction in rat pancreas, kidney and lungs but not in liver. Pancreatology, 2013;13(3):216-24.

Tsai K, Wang SS, Chen TS, Kong CW, Chang FY, Lee SD, Lu FJ. Oxidative stress: an important phenomenon with pathogenetic significance in the progression of acute pancreatitis. Gut. 1998 Jun 1;42(6):850-5.

Tsujimoto T, Tsuruzono T, Hoppo K, Matsumura Y, Yamao J, Fukui H. Effect of bromhexine hydrochloride therapy for alcoholic chronic pancreatitis. Alcoholism: Clinical and Experimental Research. 2005 Dec;29:272S-6S.

Tsutsumi S, Gotoh T, Tomisato W, Mima S, Hoshino T, Hwang HJ, Takenaka H, Tsuchiya T, Mori M, Mizushima T. Endoplasmic reticulum stress response is involved in nonsteroidal anti-inflammatory drug-induced apoptosis. Cell Death & Differentiation. 2004 Sep;11(9):1009-16.

Turner R. Screening methods in pharmacology. Elsevier; 2013 Oct 22.

Ugwah-Oguejiofor CJ, Okoli CO, Ugwah MO, Umaru ML, Ogbulie CS, Mshelia HE, Umar M, Njan AA. Acute and sub-acute toxicity of aqueous extract of aerial parts of Caralluma dalzielii NE Brown in mice and rats. Heliyon. 2019 Jan 1;5(1):e01179.

Vaidya AD, Devasagayam TP. Current status of herbal drugs in India: an overview. Journal of clinical biochemistry and nutrition. 2007;41(1):1-1.

Vincent D, Myriam D, Frédéric C, Jacques D. Fat malabsorption screening in chronic pancreatitis. American Journal of Gastroenterology. 2004 Jul 1;99(7):1350-4.

Vonlaufen A, Wilson JS, Pirola RC, Apte MV. Role of alcohol metabolism in chronic pancreatitis. Alcohol Research & Health. 2007;30(1):48.

Waldron RT, Su HY, Piplani H, Capri J, Cohn W, Whitelegge JP, Faull KF, Sakkiah S, Abrol R, Yang W, Zhou B. Ethanol induced disordering of pancreatic acinar cell endoplasmic reticulum: an ER stress/defective unfolded protein response model. Cellular and molecular gastroenterology and hepatology. 2018 Jan 1;5(4):479-97.

Walter P, Ron D. The unfolded protein response: from stress pathway to homeostatic regulation. science. 2011 Nov 25;334(6059):1081-6.

Watanabe T, Kudo M, Strober W. Immunopathogenesis of pancreatitis. Mucosal immunology. 2017 Mar;10(2):283-98.

Wehler M, Nichterlein R, Fischer B, Farnbacher M, Reulbach U, Hahn EG, Schneider T. Factors associated with health-related quality of life in chronic pancreatitis. American Journal of Gastroenterology. 2004 Jan 1;99(1):138-46.

Weniger M, Reinelt L, Neumann J, Holdt L, Ilmer M, Renz B, Hartwig W, Werner J, Bazhin AV, D'Haese JG. The analgesic effect of the mitochondria-targeted antioxidant SkQ1 in pancreatic inflammation. Oxidative medicine and cellular longevity. 2016 Jan 1;2016.

Wu D, Bai X, Lee P, Yang Y, Windsor J, Qian J. A systematic review of nsaids treatment for acute pancreatitis in animal studies and clinical trials. Clinics and Research in Hepatology and Gastroenterology: X. 2020 Jan 1;1:100002.

Wu J, Luo X, Yan LJ. Two dimensional blue native/SDS-PAGE to identify mitochondrial complex I subunits modified by 4-hydroxynonenal (HNE). Front Physiol, 2015; 6:98.

Wu L, Cai B, Zheng S, Liu X, Cai H, Li H. Effect of emodin on endoplasmic reticulum stress in rats with severe acute pancreatitis. Inflammation. 2013 Oct 1;36(5):1020-9.

Xue J, Li R, Zhao X, Ma C, Lv X, Liu L, Liu P. Morusin induces paraptosis-like cell death through mitochondrial calcium overload and dysfunction in epithelial ovarian cancer. Chemico-biological interactions. 2018 Mar 1;283:59-74.

Yang R, Yuan BC, Ma YS, Zhou S, Liu Y. The anti-inflammatory activity of licorice, a widely used Chinese herb. Pharmaceutical biology. 2017 Jan 1;55(1):5-18.

Yang ZW, Meng XX, Xu P. Central role of neutrophil in the pathogenesis of severe acute pancreatitis. Journal of cellular and molecular medicine. 2015 Nov;19(11):2513-20.

Yao W, Maitra A, Ying H. Recent insights into the biology of pancreatic cancer. EBioMedicine. 2020 Mar 1;53:102655.

Yu JH, Lim JW, Namkung W, Kim H, Kim KH. Suppression of cerulein-induced cytokine expression by antioxidants in pancreatic acinar cells. Laboratory investigation. 2002 Oct;82(10):1359-68.

Yu K, Chen F, Li C. Absorption, disposition, and pharmacokinetics of saponins from Chinese medicinal herbs: what do we know and what do we need to know more?. Current drug metabolism. 2012 Jun 1;13(5):577-98.

Yuet Ping K, Darah I, Chen Y, Sreeramanan S, Sasidharan S. Acute and subchronic toxicity study of Euphorbia hirta L. methanol extract in rats. BioMed research international. 2013; 2013: 182064.

Zang Q, Maass DL, White J, Horton JW. Cardiac mitochondrial damage and loss of ROS defense after burn injury: the beneficial effects of antioxidant therapy. J Appl Physiol, 2007; 102(1):103-12.

Zargari-Samadnejad A, Mehrvarz S, Allizadeh-Naeini S, Tanideh N. Healing effect of Licorice extract in acetic acid-induced ulcerative colitis in rat. Research in Pharmaceutical Sciences. 2012 Sep 2;7(5):837.

Zhao Q, Zhang H, Huang J, Yu H, Li J, Che Q, Sun Y, Jin Y, Wu J. Melatonin attenuates the inflammatory response via inhibiting the C/EBP homologous protein-mediated pathway in taurocholate-induced acute pancreatitis. International Journal of Molecular Medicine. 2018 Dec 1;42(6):3513-21.

Zhao X, Lang R, Zhang Z, Zhao W, Ji Z, Tan H, Zhou X. Exploring and validating the clinical risk factors for pancreatic cancer in chronic pancreatitis patients using electronic medical records datasets: three cohorts comprising 2,960 patients. Translational Cancer Research. 2020 Feb 1;9(2):629-38.

Zheng D, Liwinski T, Elinav E. Inflammasome activation and regulation: toward a better understanding of complex mechanisms. Cell discovery. 2020 Jun 9;6(1):1-22.

Zhou L, Tan JH, Cao RC, Xu J, Chen XM, Qi ZC, Zhou SY, Li SB, Mo QX, Li ZW, Zhang GW. ATF6 regulates the development of chronic pancreatitis by inducing p53-mediated apoptosis. Cell death & disease. 2019 Sep10;10(9):1-2.

Zhou R, Yazdi AS, Menu P, Tschopp J. A role for mitochondria in NLRP3 inflammasome activation. Nature, 2011;469(7329):221-5.

Zinszner H, Kuroda M, Wang X, Batchvarova N, Lightfoot RT, Remotti H, Stevens JL, Ron D. CHOP is implicated in programmed cell death in response to impaired function of the endoplasmic reticulum. Genes & development. 1998 Apr 1;12(7):982-95.

10. PUBLICATIONS

1. Srikantam S, Arumugam G. Hydroalcoholic extract of licorice (Glycyrrhiza glabra L.) root attenuates ethanol and cerulein induced pancreatitis in rats. Asian Pacific Journal of Tropical Biomedicine. 2019 Oct 1;9(10):424.

2. Srikantam S, Arumugam G. Glycyrrhizin modulates ER stress-induced UPR and concomitant mitochondrial dysfunction and activation of NF-κB in alcohol and cerulein-induced pancreatitis in rats. Journal of Applied Pharmaceutical Science. 2021 Mar;11(03):130-40.

11. CONFERENCES ATTENDED

1. Presented a paper entitled "Phytochemical profiling of hydroalcoholic root extract of Glycyrrhiza glabra L. and investigation of its protective effect against ethanol and cerulein-induced chronic pancreatitis-A study in male albino Wistar rats." held on 30 and 31 July 2018, at Dr. MGR-Janaki Arts and Science College for Women, Chennai.

2. Presented a paper entitled "A study on ER stress and mitochondrial dysfunctions in alcohol-cerulein induced chronic pancreatitis in rats-Modulating effect of *Glycyrrhiza glabra* L.(Adhimadhuram)." held on 28th September 2018, at Central Council for Research in Siddha(CCRS), Chennai.

3. Presented a paper entitled "Evaluation of pancreato-protective effect of licorice (Glycyrrhiza glabra L.) root extract against ethanol and cerulein-induced chronic pancreatitis in rats" held on 4th and 5th March 2020, at Dr. Ambedkar Government Arts College, Chennai.

Wolters Kluwer
Medknow
IF: 1.59
ISSN 2221-1691(Print)
ISSN 2588-9222(Online)
CODEN APJTC7

Asian Pacific Journal of Tropical Biomedicine

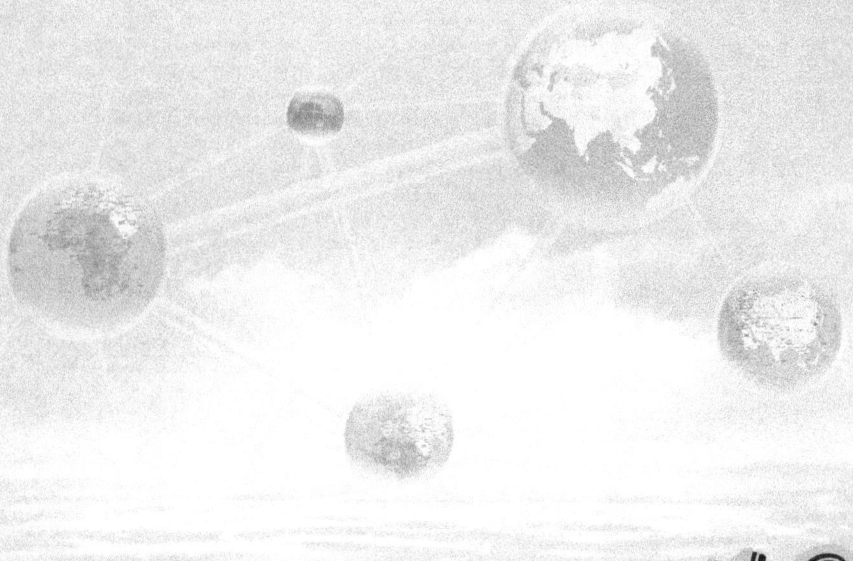

10
2019
ISSN 2221-1691
10 >
772221 169194
Vol 9 No 10 Oct

Original Article

Asian Pacific Journal of Tropical Biomedicine

journal homepage: www.apjtb.org

doi: 10.4103/2221-1691.269524

Impact factor: 1.59

Hydroalcoholic extract of licorice (*Glycyrrhiza glabra* L.) root attenuates ethanol and cerulein induced pancreatitis in rats

Sarmishta Srikantam[1], Geetha Arumugam[2]✉

[1]*Department of Biochemistry, Bharathi Women's College, Broadway, Chennai, India*

[2]*Dr. Ambedkar Government Arts College, Vyasarpadi, Chennai, India*

ARTICLE INFO

Article history:
Received 8 April 2019
Revision 17 May 2019
Accepted 12 September 2019
Available online 24 October 2019

Keywords:
Pancreatitis
ROS
Inflammation
Glycyrrhiza glabra
HPLC
GC-MS

ABSTRACT

Objective: To evaluate the therapeutic potential of hydroalcoholic extract of licorice root against ethanol and cerulein induced chronic pancreatitis in rats.

Methods: The phytochemical profile of hydroalcoholic extract of licorice root was determined by high performance liquid chromatography (HPLC) and gas chromatography coupled to mass spectrometry (GC-MS). Chronic pancreatitis was induced in male albino Wistar rats by feeding them a diet containing ethanol (0%-36% of total calories) for 4 weeks and cerulein (20 μg/kg b.wt, i.p.) thrice a week for 3 weeks. Lipase and amylase in serum, lipid peroxides and antioxidants including reduced glutathione, glutathione peroxidase, superoxide dismutase and catalase in pancreas were determined. Inflammatory response was measured by myeloperoxidase in the pancreas, caspase-1 and the concentrations of IL-1β and IL-18 in serum. Moreover, histological evaluation of the pancreas and liver was carried out.

Results: Different flavonoids and saponins were identified in the hydroalcoholic extract of licorice root through HPLC and GC-MS. A marked increase in the levels of serum lipase, amylase, lipid peroxides, caspase-1, myeloperoxidase, IL-1β, and IL-18 and a marked decrease in the levels of antioxidants were observed after ethanol and cerulein administration. Treatment with hydroalcoholic extract of licorice root attenuated these changes. In addition, histological observation confirmed the protective effect of the extract in the pancreas and liver against inflammatory changes induced by ethanol and cerulein.

Conclusions: The licorice root extract attenuates ethanol and cerulein induced pancreatitis in rats probably due to its antioxidant phytonutrients since ethanol and cerulein-induced production of reactive oxygen species contributes to severe inflammation in the pancreas.

1. Introduction

The pancreas consists of acinar and islet cells which synthesize and secrete digestive enzymes and hormones, respectively. Acute or chronic pancreatitis is characterized by inflammatory reactions that result in the premature intracellular or interstitial activation of trypsinogen causing pancreatic auto-digestion. Acute pancreatitis (AP) is of sudden onset and short duration. Recurrent AP can lead to chronic pancreatitis (CP) which is a progressive inflammatory and fibrotic disease. It develops gradually and worsens over time, resulting in the irreversible weakening of the pancreas, causing pancreatic exocrine and endocrine insufficiencies. CP is a known

✉Corresponding author: Dr. A. Geetha, Dr. Ambedkar Government Arts College Vyasarpadi, Chennai – 600 039, Tamilnadu, India.
Tel: +91-94449 02506, +91-790431 6378
E-mail: geethav21@yahoo.co.in

How to cite this article: Srikantam S, Arumugam G. Hydroalcoholic extract of licorice (*Glycyrrhiza glabra* L.) root attenuates ethanol and cerulein induced pancreatitis in rats. Asian Pac J Trop Biomed 2019; 9(10): 424-433.

risk factor for pancreatic adenocarcinoma.

CP is associated with severe abdominal pain, maldigestion, malabsorption, steatorrhea, and weight loss. Alcohol abuse, gallstone-related diseases and recurrent AP are found to be the major causes of CP. Alcohol abuse is the primary cause of CP, accounting for nearly 70%–80% of all cases[1]. Alcoholic chronic pancreatitis which affects the quality of life was previously more prevalent in developed countries, but is now increasing worldwide due to increased alcohol consumption[2].

Rats, when chronically administered ethanol, have an increased susceptibility to AP induced by cerulein. Cerulein, an analogue of cholecystokinin, elicits pancreatic injury by hyperstimulation of the exocrine pancreas. The key features of human alcoholic CP are reproduced in the rat with ethanol and repeated doses of cerulein[3]. In pancreatic acinar cells, local inflammation is thus initiated by the release of inflammatory mediators called cytokines (IL-1 β, IL-6, IL-10 and TNF-α) and chemokines. TNF-α is a potent activator of NF-κB, a pro-inflammatory transcription factor. The initial inflammatory process leads to the recruitment of innate immune cells such as neutrophils and macrophages towards the site of injury. These immune cells play a critical role in the pathogenesis of pancreatitis. Neutrophils increase disease severity by the production of reactive oxygen species (ROS)[4]. These infiltrating cells along with injured acinar cells, in turn, produce more cytokines and chemokines increasing inflammatory response in the pancreas. CP also results in oxidative stress which amplifies the inflammatory process.

Pancreatic acinar cells are known to metabolize ethanol. Ethanol-induced toxicity is mediated mostly through the oxidative and non-oxidative metabolism of ethanol. In oxidative metabolism, alcohol dehydrogenase (ADH) oxidizes ethanol to acetaldehyde followed by conversion of acetaldehyde to acetate by aldehyde dehydrogenase (ALDH), specifically localized in the mitochondrion. Depletion of oxidized nicotinamide adenine dinucleotide (NAD^+) and accumulation of reduced nicotinamide adenine dinucleotide (NADH) take place, as both ADH and ALDH consume NAD^+, producing NADH. Oxidative metabolism of ethanol to acetaldehyde by CYP2E1 produces excessive ROS which also activates NF-κB which is highly ROS sensitive. In non-oxidative metabolism, fatty acid ethyl ester (FAEE) synthase converts ethanol to FAEE. Thus, ethanol metabolism results in accumulation of acetaldehyde, acetate, NADH and FAEE, as well as changes in cellular and mitochondrial NAD^+ and NADH levels. FAEEs are known to generate a sustained increase in intracellular calcium and subsequent mitochondrial injury, in turn contributing to oxidative stress[5].

Cerulein binds to a G-protein coupled receptor called cholecystokinin receptor on the pancreatic acinar cell membrane and activates phospholipase C and inositol triphosphate-dependent calcium release from the endoplasmic reticulum. This can activate NADPH oxidase which produces ROS, which can disturb the integrity of mitochondria by causing mitochondrial dysfunction. ROS can also cause cytokine signalling through NF-κB pathway[6]. Increased ROS also results in the oxidation of lipids and proteins and disruption of the pancreatic cell membrane. ROS, proteases and growth factors released by neutrophils and macrophages cause tissue destruction, as well as fibroblast proliferation[7].

The stroma of the pancreas has a clinically important cell type called pancreatic stellate cells (PSCs). In the pancreas, PSCs maintain normal tissue architecture through the synthesis and degradation of extracellular matrix proteins (like collagen). Various pathophysiological changes following pancreatic injury transform quiescent stellate cells into myofibroblast-like cells which actively proliferate and produce more extracellular matrix proteins leading to fibrosis observed in CP. Many scientific reports explained that damage to the pancreatic tissue caused by ethanol and its metabolite acetaldehyde (through MAP kinase pathway), ROS and pro-inflammatory cytokines causes the activation of PSCs. Release of growth factors such as the platelet-derived growth factor, transforming growth factors (TGF-β) secreted by infiltrating cells (monocytes, macrophages) also leads to persistent activation of PSCs[8]. Deng *et al* has reported that chronic ethanol administration increases fibrosis formation in response to cerulein-induced pancreatitis in rats and is highly driven by anti-inflammatory responses to pancreatic injury and/or chronic oxidative stress. So, the recruitment of inflammatory cells provides cytokine signals for PSC activation and fibrosis formation in CP[3].

The major event responsible for the disease severity, progression and cell death in pancreatitis is NF-κB activation. NF-κB mediated pathway is central inflammatory pathway that operates in pancreatitis. Damage associated molecular patterns (DAMPs) released from dead and dying pancreatic acinar cells, ROS, acetaldehyde and FAEEs from ethanol metabolism were reported to activate NF-κB in CP. Ethanol also sensitizes pancreas to the inflammatory response through protein kinase C-mediated pathway of NF-κB activation[9]. Cerulein causes NF-κB activation through NADPH oxidase that produces ROS. NF-κB is kept inactive in the cytoplasm through sequestration in complexes with the inhibitor of NF-κB (IκB) proteins. The sequestration prevents NF-κB migration into the nucleus, its binding to DNA and transcriptional activation. In response to stimuli, the IκBs are phosphorylated on specific serine residues by IκB kinases, resulting in IκB ubiquitylation and proteasome-mediated degradation. This allows nuclear translocation of NF-κB, to mediate the expression of cytokines. ROS generated in response to ethanol and cerulein could activate IκB kinase and NF-κB[6]. Furthermore, ethanol treatment augments the cerulein-induced activation of NF-κB.

Pancreatic acinar cell death releases endogenous molecules of the host DAMPs, into the extracellular space that triggers inflammation. Acinar cells and recruited inflammatory cells have pattern recognition receptors to recognise DAMPs. DAMPs mediate the assembly and activation of receptor complexes called inflammasomes. Signalling through pattern recognition receptors like toll like receptor 4 and 9 results in activation of NF-κB facilitated inflammasome. Different types of inflammasomes are characterized in different organs. NLRP3 is one such inflammasome activated in pancreas in response to cell injury by endogenous and exogenous sources. Activation of NLRP3 inflammasome releases active form of caspase-1, a cytosolic protease which converts pro-

IL-1 β and pro-IL-18 to active IL-1 β and IL-18, serving a central role in the inflammatory response[10]. Oxidative stress and its constant companion persistent inflammation, play critical roles in the pathogenesis of CP and its many complications.

Most therapies center on pain relief with non-steroidal anti-inflammatory drugs (NSAIDs) and management of exocrine and endocrine shortages by supportive therapy. But long-term treatment with NSAIDs can induce pain tolerance, addiction and severe side effects. As there is no single modality treatment approach for CP, it is essential to identify effective and less toxic natural compounds.

Natural products play a crucial role in modern drug development. Many studies reported that plant extracts or plant secondary metabolites such as phenolic compounds, saponins and flavonoids show anti-inflammatory activity. They control the levels of various inflammatory cytokines and their most important regulator, nuclear factor NF-κB[11]. To exploit such properties, the present study focused on an effective and potential ayurvedic medicinal herb, *Glycyrrhiza glabra* Linn. (*G. glabra*). It is a perennial herb of the pea family (Fabaceae) found widely in Asia and the Mediterranean region. It is commonly known as 'yastimadhu' or licorice. Wide spread use of licorice as demulcent, expectorant and in ulcer healing is well documented in traditions from ancient Assyrian, Egyptian, Chinese and Indian cultures[12].

Licorice roots have been shown to possess anti-inflammatory, anti-oxidative, anti-viral and expectorant properties. They are also found effective in increasing the detoxification capacity of the liver. Phytochemically, licorice roots have shown to contain triterpene saponins, flavonoids, coumarins and phytosterols. The biologically-active components of licorice are glycyrrhizic acid, liquiritin, glabridin and liquiritigenin[13].

This study was conducted to evaluate whether licorice root extract can ameliorate oxidative stress and alter the levels of cytokines responsible for inflammation in the pancreas of male albino Wistar rats administered ethanol and cerulein.

2. Materials and methods

2.1. Chemicals

ELISA kits for caspase-1 and IL-1 β were purchased from Abcam, ELISA kit for IL-18 purchased was from Invitrogen BioServices, India. All the other chemicals and solvents used for the analysis were of analytical grade and were purchased from Merck, India.

2.2. Preparation of plant extract

The licorice roots were bought from the local market (Chennai) and authenticated by Dr. P. Jayaraman, Taxonomist, Plant Anatomy Research Centre, Chennai, Tamilnadu (specimen no. PARC/2016/3303). Surface cleaned roots were shade-dried, pulverized and macerated with 70% ethanol (in water) at room temperature. Maceration was carried out by soaking the pulverized roots in 70% ethanol for 3 d with frequent agitation in a shaker. Then the mixture was strained, pressed and soaked again in ethanol. The maceration step was repeated 3-4 times[14]. Finally, the combined filtrate was clarified by filtration using Whatmann no.1 filter paper, semi air-dried and lyophilized to gain the hydroalcoholic extract of licorice root and stored at 4 ℃ until further analysis. The yield was 12% w/w.

2.3. High performance liquid chromatography (HPLC) analysis of hydroalcoholic extract of licorice root

HPLC analysis was carried out on Shimadzu HPLC CLASS-VP™ series equipped with 2489 UV/Visible detector for the identification and quantitative determination of phytochemicals in hydroalcoholic extract of licorice root. EZChrom Elite Data System was used for data acquisition, processing and control of HPLC and report generation.

2.3.1. Identification and quantification of flavonoids

About 10 g of hydroalcoholic extract of licorice root was refluxed with the extraction solvent - alcohol, water and hydrochloric acid mixture (50:20:8) - on a hot water bath for 135 min (to hydrolyse glycosides to aglycones), then decanted and sonicated for 30 min using methanol. The contents were filtered and diluted to 100 mL with methanol. Quercetin, kaempferol, isorhamnetin, galangin, luteolin, rutin and thymoquinone served as the reference standards. The mobile phase used was a mixture of methanol, water, and phosphoric acid (100:100:1). The samples were run on symmetry C18 column [100 Å pore size, 3.5 μm, 4.6 mm × 250 mm (product no. WAT200632)] with a flow rate of 1.5 mL per minute. Isocratically eluted compounds were detected by UV detector at 270 nm. By matching the retention time and their spectral characteristics against those of the standards, the flavonoids were identified in hydroalcoholic extract of licorice root.

2.3.2. Identification and quantification of saponins

Equal volumes of glycyrrhizin standard and sample (20 μL) were separately injected into the chromatograph and the separation was carried out by isocratic elution. Methanol-water-acetic acid mixture (60:34:6) was the mobile phase used. The flow rate was 1 mL/min through a C-18 reverse phase column. Measurement of UV absorbance was done at 254 nm[15]. By matching the retention time and the spectral characteristics against that of the standard, a saponin was identified in hydroalcoholic extract of licorice root.

2.4. Phytochemical screening by gas chromatography coupled to mass spectrometry (GC-MS)

Hydroalcoholic extract of licorice root was subjected to GC-MS analysis on Agilent 6890N gas chromatograph with HP-5MS column, coupled to a mass spectrometer JEOL GC-MATE Ⅱ in the electron ionization mode with ionization voltage set to 70 eV. The mass spectral scan range of the mass analyser was set to 50-600 amu. Carrier gas used was helium, at a constant flow of 1 mL/min. The GC-oven was set at a ramp rate from 50 ℃-250 ℃ at 10 ℃/min.

Compounds were identified using NIST database (National Institute of Standards and Technology).

2.5. Animals

Male albino Wistar rats weighing 175-200 g were maintained on a 12-hour light-dark cycle at 25 ℃, humidity between 60% and 70%. The rats were housed in polyethylene cages, and given free access to standard rat chow pellets and water during the acclimatization period. Institutional Animal Ethics Committee approved the experimental protocol (XIX/VELS/PCOL/06/2000/CPCSEA/IAEC/03.10.2016).

2.6. Induction of chronic pancreatitis using ethanol and cerulein

After the acclimatization for 1 week, rats were randomly assigned into 4 groups (6 rats in each group). Group 1 (control) and 2 (100 mg/kg body weight of hydroalcoholic extract of licorice root) rats were fed standard rat chow and water *ad libitum* for 5 weeks. Group 3 (ethanol + cerulein) and 4 (ethanol + cerulein + 100 mg/kg body weight of hydroalcoholic extract of licorice root) were fed an isocalorically adjusted diet containing ethanol (0%-36% of total calories) for 4 weeks and subjected to intraperitoneal injection of cerulein (20 μg/kg body weight) 3 times a week for the last three weeks[3]. Group 2 and 4 rats received 100 mg/kg body weight of hydroalcoholic extract of licorice root orally from the third week onwards. Initially, a dose-response study was conducted with different concentrations (25, 50, 100 and 200 mg/kg body weight) of hydroalcoholic extract of licorice root and a dose of 100 mg/kg body weight, which gave the maximum anti-inflammatory activity against pancreatitis was selected for further study.

After 5 weeks, all the animals were fasted overnight, anesthetized using diethyl ether and euthanized by cervical decapitation. Immediately, blood was collected, the serum separated and stored at 4 ℃ until further analyses. Pancreas and liver were removed immediately. A part of these organs from each rat was fixed in 10% formal saline for 24 h and subjected to processing for histopathological examinations.

2.7. Preparation of tissue homogenate

The isolated pancreas was washed with ice cold saline and homogenized in 0.1 M Tris HCl buffer (pH 7.4) at low temperature. The supernatant was used to determine protein, reduced glutathione (GSH), lipid peroxides and the antioxidant enzymes-superoxide dismutase (SOD), catalase (CAT) and glutathione peroxidase (GPx).

2.8. Biochemical investigations

2.8.1. Determination of serum lipase and serum amylase activity

The activity of lipase in serum was assayed according to the method of Lowry and Tinsley[16]. The lipolysis reaction was initiated with the addition of serum in 25 mL olive oil/triton-emulsion as substrate. About 0.3 mL subsamples of the reaction mixture were taken at pre-determined intervals and used for the assay of liberated free fatty acids spectrophotometrically at 715 nm. The activity of the enzyme was expressed as IU/L.

According to the method of Gomori[17], the enzyme activity was determined by measuring the maltose liberated from the starch (substrate) using Lugol's iodine solution. The color intensity was measured spectrophotometrically at 640 nm and the enzyme activity was expressed as IU/L.

2.8.2. Estimation of protein

The protein content of pancreatic homogenate was measured according to the method of Bradford[18] and was used to calculate the specific activities of enzymes.

2.8.3. Estimation of GSH and antioxidant enzymes

GSH level was determined by the method of Moron *et al*[19] and expressed as mg/g protein. GPx was assayed by the method of Flohe and Gunzler[20]. The activity of GPx was expressed as nM of glutathione oxidized/min/mg protein. SOD activity was measured according to the method of Kakkar *et al*[21]. The assay is based on the inhibition of formation of NADH-phenazine-methosulfate nitroblue tetrazolium formazan. The color developed was extracted with *n*-butanol and measured at 560 nm. CAT activity was defined as the amount of enzyme required to decompose 1 μM of H_2O_2 per min. Decomposition of H_2O_2 in the presence of CAT was kinetically measured at 240 nm.The enzyme activity was expressed as μM of H_2O_2 consumed/min/mg protein[22].

2.8.4. Estimation of lipid peroxides

Malondialdehyde (MDA) and 4-hydroxynonenal (4-HNE) are the main products of lipid peroxidation. MDA is a major reactive aldehyde resulting from peroxidation of membrane lipids. TBARS assay was used to determine MDA level[23] and the value was expressed as nM/mg tissue protein.

To estimate 4-HNE, the pancreatic homogenate was allowed to react with 2,4-dinitrophenylhydrazine, mixed thoroughly and set aside for 1 h to react with 4-HNE in the sample. Then the formed adduct of 4-HNE and DNPH was extracted thrice with hexane and evaporated to dryness at 40 ℃. After cooling, 1 mL methanol was added to the residue and the absorbance read at 350 nm spectrophotometrically.

2.8.5. Estimation of inflammatory markers

Myeloperoxidase (MPO), IL-1β, IL-18 and caspase-1 are the major markers of pancreatic inflammation. MPO was extracted from homogenized tissue and activity was measured according to the method of Bradley *et al*[24]. The change in absorbance after adding the reagents [50 mM potassium phosphate buffer (pH 6.0) containing 0.167 mg/mL o-dianisidine dihydrochloride and 0.000 5% hydrogen peroxide] was measured at 460 nm for 4 min using UV-visible spectrophotometer and expressed as units/mg protein. The assay of IL-1β was performed according to the manual of Rat IL-1β ELISA Kit (ab100767) and the activity was expressed as pg/mL. The assay of IL-18 was carried out according to the manual of Rat IL-18 ELISA Kit (KRC2341) and the activity was expressed as pg/mL.The assay of caspase-1 was performed in undiluted serum and suitably diluted pancreatic tissue homogenate according to the procedure shown in caspase-1 activity assay kit (ab39470). The assay is based on spectrophotometric detection of the chromophore *p*-nitroanilide (*p*-NA) derived from the labeled substrate YVAD-*p*-NA by the activity of caspase-1 present in the sources.

2.9. Histopathological examinations

The fixative was washed from formalin-fixed pancreas and liver tissue samples, dehydrated through a graded series of alcohol, cleaned in methyl benzoate and embedded in paraffin wax. The paraffin-embedded tissue samples were then sectioned (5 μm), stained with hematoxylin and eosin. The slides were then observed under light microscope at 400x magnification.

2.10. Statistical analysis

Data were analysed by the statistics software package (SPSS for Windows v.10). The statistical significance of mean values between different groups was determined by one-way ANOVA with *post hoc* Bonferroni test and P value < 0.05 was considered significant.

3. Results

3.1. HPLC analysis of hydroalcoholic extract of licorice root

3.1.1. Identification and quantification of flavonoids

HPLC-UV chromatogram of the flavonoids in hydroalcoholic extract of licorice root showed the presence of four major peaks at 270 nm with the retention times of 4.527, 11.310, 16.890 and 40.010 min, respectively (Figure 1B). The peaks were identified as rutin, luteolin, thymoquinone and galangin at a concentration of 0.9 mg/g, 0.6 mg/g, 0.5 mg/g, and 1.3 mg/g, respectively. Compounds were confirmed through the comparison of their retention times with those of the standards (Figure 1A).

3.1.2. Identification and quantification of saponins

Figure 1D displays the HPLC-UV chromatogram of saponins of hydroalcoholic extract of licorice root. A peak was found at 254 nm with the retention time of 31.37 min. It was confirmed to be glycyrrhizin by matching the retention time and spectral characteristics with that of glycyrrhizin standard at different concentrations (Figure 1C). Concentration of glycyrrhizin was calculated through a calibration graph and found to be 0.02 mg/g.

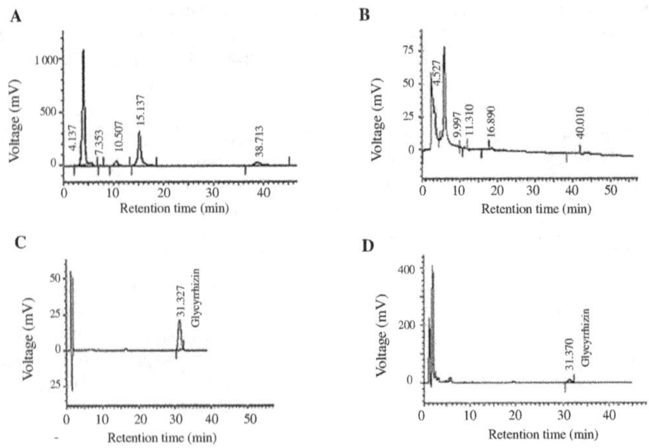

Figure 1. HPLC chromatogram of (A) flavanoid standards, RT 4.137 =rutin; RT 10.507=luteolin; RT 15.137=thymoquinone; RT 38.713=galangin; (B) flavonoids detected in hydroalcoholic extract of licorice root, RT 4.527=rutin; RT 11.310=luteolin; RT 16.890=thymoquinone; RT 40.010=galangin; (C) saponin standard, glycyrrhizin; (D) saponins detected in hydroalcoholic extract of licorice root. RT: retention time in min.

Table 1. Phytochemicals identified in hydroalcoholic extract of licorice root by GC-MS.

RT (min)	Name of the compound	Molecular formula*	Molecular weight* (g/mol)	Nature of the compound*	Bioactivity†
9.10	3-Hydroxy-3',4',5,7-tetramethoxyflavone	$C_{19}H_{18}O_7$	358.3	Flavone	Protector against lipid peroxidation, antiviral, and anti-proliferative
9.70	4H-1-Benzopyran-4-one,5,7-bis(acetyloxy)-2-[4-(acetyloxy)-3-methoxyphenyl]-3,6-dimethoxy-(jaceidin triacetate)	$C_{24}H_{22}O_{11}$	486.4	Flavone	Antibacterial
10.37	Undecane/ hendecane	$C_{11}H_{24}$	156.3	Alkane hydrocarbon	-

*PubChem, Human Metabolome Database; †science.gov, Dr. Duke's Phytochemical and Ethnobotanical Database. RT: retention time.

3.2. Phytochemical screening by GC–MS

Three compounds were detected in hydroalcoholic extract of licorice root by GC-MS analysis: 3-hydroxy-3',4',5,7-tetramethoxyflavone, jaceidin triacetate and undecane (Table 1). The GC-MS chromatogram of hydroalcoholic extract of licorice root was shown in supplementary Figure 1.

3.3. Effect of hydroalcoholic extract of licorice root on pancreatitis marker levels

Table 2 shows the activity levels of serum lipase and serum amylase in all experimental groups. Rats administered ethanol and cerulein showed significant elevation in the activity when compared to the control ($P < 0.05$). Serum levels of these markers reverted towards normal in rats treated with hydroalcoholic extract of licorice root ($P < 0.05$). Rats fed normal diet as well as hydroalcoholic extract of licorice root alone showed normal enzyme activities.

3.4. Effect of hydroalcoholic extract of licorice root on antioxidant parameters

Activities of GSH, GPx, SOD, CAT in all the groups are presented in Table 3. Their activities decreased significantly in pancreatitis-induced rats compared to the control. No significant changes were observed in the rats treated with hydroalcoholic extract of licorice root alone in comparison with the control. In rats administered ethanol and cerulein as well as hydroalcoholic extract of licorice root, the levels of these cellular antioxidants increased.

Table 2. Effect of hydroalcoholic extract of licorice root (HAELR) on lipase and amylase levels (IU/L).

Groups	Lipase	Amylase
Control	1.73±0.23	1 832.21±218.03
HAELR	1.69±0.18	1 714.02±222.82
EtOH + Cerulein	4.16±0.42*	3 872.47±398.47*
EtOH + Cerulein + HAELR	2.27±0.28#	2 298.78±264.30#

Data were analysed by one-way ANOVA followed by *post–hoc* Bonferroni test. Values are expressed as mean ± SD of six rats in each group. EtOH: ethanol. Statistical significance was calculated by comparing Control *vs.* EtOH + Cerulein; EtOH + Cerulein *vs.* EtOH + Cerulein +HAELR; *P=0.00 and #P<0.05.

3.5. Effect of hydroalcoholic extract of licorice root on lipid peroxidation

Levels of lipid peroxides including TBARS (MDA) and 4-HNE are presented in Table 4. An increase in the levels of lipid peroxidation products was found in the group administered ethanol and cerulein compared to the control. Treatment with hydroalcoholic extract of licorice root markedly reduced the levels of TBARS and 4-HNE. Levels of TBARS and 4-HNE showed no significant change in the rats treated with hydroalcoholic extract of licorice root alone.

3.6. Effect of hydroalcoholic extract of licorice root on inflammatory markers

The levels of MPO, caspase-1, IL-1β and IL-18 in the experimental rats are presented in Table 5. A significant increase in the levels of these inflammatory markers was observed in pancreatitis-induced rats compared to the control. These levels reduced significantly in rats co-administered hydroalcoholic extract of licorice root. There were no significant changes in the levels of inflammatory markers in the group treated with hydroalcoholic extract of licorice root alone.

3.7. Histopathological observations

Figure 2 and Figure 3 illustrate the photomicrographs of pancreas and liver from all the experimental groups, respectively. Pancreatic and liver sections from the control and the group treated with hydroalcoholic extract of licorice root alone showed normal tissue architecture without any abnormal activity (Figure 2A, Figure 2B and Figure 3A, Figure 3B). Sections of the pancreas from ethanol and cerulein administered group showed neutrophil infiltration and fibrotic changes (Figure 2C). Its liver section also showed tissue infiltration with neutrophils (Figure 3C). Tissue architecture of pancreas (Figure 2D) and liver (Figure 3D) of pancreatitis-induced rats co-administered hydroalcoholic extract of licorice root at 100 mg/kg was improved.

Table 3. Effect of hydroalcoholic extract of licorice root (HAELR) on antioxidant parameters.

Groups	GSH (mg/g protein)	GPx (nM GSH oxidized/min/mg protein)	SOD (Units/mg protein)	CAT (μM of H_2O_2 consumed/min/mg protein)
Control	56.20±6.57	80.20±10.34	13.50±1.53	105.20±13.00
HAELR	55.30±6.85	79.80±9.57	13.00±1.67	103.60±11.95
EtOH + Cerulein	21.40±3.18*	48.80±6.99*	6.90±0.96*	70.90±10.45*
EtOH + Cerulein + HAELR	44.50±6.43#	68.20±8.72#	11.20±1.40#	97.40±10.90#

Data were analysed by one-way ANOVA followed by *post–hoc* Bonferroni test. Values are expressed as mean ± SD of six rats in each group. GSH: glutathione; GPx: glutathione peroxidase; SOD: superoxide dismutase; CAT: catalase; EtOH: ethanol. Statistical significance was calculated by comparing Control *vs.* EtOH + Cerulein; EtOH + Cerulein *vs.* EtOH + Cerulein +HAELR; *P=0.00 and #P<0.05.

Table 4. Effect of hydroalcoholic extract of licorice root (HAELR) on lipid peroxidation.

Groups	TBARS (MDA) (nM/mg protein)	4-HNE (μM/g protein)
Control	29.80±3.14	1.98±0.22
HAELR	30.70±3.77	2.12±0.27
EtOH + Cerulein	51.10±5.57*	8.30±0.84*
EtOH + Cerulein + HAELR	33.90±4.17#	4.89±0.59#

Data were analysed by one-way ANOVA followed by *post-hoc* Bonferroni test. Values are expressed as mean ± SD of six rats in each group. TBARS: thiobarbituric acid-reacting substances; MDA: Malondialdehyde; 4-HNE: 4-hydroxynonenal; EtOH: ethanol. Statistical significance was calculated by comparing Control *vs.* EtOH + Cerulein; EtOH + Cerulein *vs.* EtOH + Cerulein +HAELR; *P=0.00 and #P<0.05.

4. Discussion

In the present investigation, hydroalcoholic extract of licorice root was evaluated for its ameliorating effect on pancreatic inflammation using rat model with ethanol and cerulein-induced pancreatitis. Recurrent AP induced by cerulein promotes chronic changes in the pancreas. Ethanol acts as a progression factor to trigger inflammatory and immune responses[3]. Chronic ethanol administration increases the pancreatic content of cathepsin B, a lysosomal cysteine protease that causes intrapancreatic activation of trypsinogen leading to the autodigestion of pancreas. Subsequent cell injury is mediated by the activated proteases. Ethanol lessens the recovery from AP and sensitizes pancreas to chronic injury through toxic effects of its metabolites on acinar cells, oxidative stress and promoting activation of PSCs, the major fibrogenic cells in the pancreas. The innate immune response of these cells is important in the induction of pancreatic inflammation[25].

As mentioned earlier, pancreatic acinar cells are the major sites of ethanol metabolism. Oxidative metabolism of ethanol by CYP2E1 produces toxic aldehydes that lead to increased ROS, triggering oxidative stress and activation of NF-κB. When ROS production overwhelms the antioxidant defence, the uncontrolled ROS generation causes cellular injury and dysfunction. NF-κB is involved in regulating the gene expression of inflammatory molecules including chemokine and cytokines like TNF-α[26]. NF-κB was shown to be activated by cerulein in rat acinar cells making it the best animal model of experimental pancreatitis. Non-oxidative ethanol metabolism involves formation of FAEE that disrupts the acinar cell membrane.

A wide range of phytoconstituents proved their role in the modulation of inflammatory response and their potency as oxidative stress modulators. Many phytonutrients work by inhibiting the inflammatory pathways as satisfactorily as NSAIDs but with less toxicity. Therefore, the focus of this investigation is on novel natural products which may shift the treatment paradigm for CP.

G. glabra, a flavoring herb, is known for its medicinal properties in the indigenous system of Ayurvedic medicine. It is also known that compounds with antioxidant properties may exert anti-inflammatory effects. Based on the previous evidences[27,28], it is hypothesized that hydroalcoholic extract of licorice root could be pancreato-protective and is investigated *in vivo*.

GC/MS is the most robust tool for plant metabolite profiling and is adopted for identifying the metabolites in hydroalcoholic extract of licorice root. Inspection of results lead to the detection of rare flavonoids such as 3-hydroxy-3',4',5,7-tetramethoxyflavone which is reported to be an excellent protector against lipid peroxidation. The 3-OH group and the electron presenting substituents like OH/-OCH3 groups at positions 5 and 7 are important for its antioxidant activity[29]. The other rare flavonoid[30] detected was jaceidin triacetate with modest antioxidative activity[31]. These compounds might contribute to the antioxidant nature of licorice roots and could have attenuated oxidative stress in pancreas.

HPLC-UV analysis showed the presence of flavonoids like rutin, quercetin and luteolin; quinones like thymoquinone; saponins like glycyrrhizin in hydroalcoholic extract of licorice root. The presence of glycyrrhizin, a pentacyclic triterpenic saponin which is anti-inflammatory[32] was also confirmed.

Both serum lipase and amylase levels were increased in pancreatitis-induced rats. These enzyme levels were reverted towards normal in rats co-administered hydroalcoholic extract of licorice root, highlighting the pancreato-protective effect of the extract. In a similar study, Abed *et al* reported that the increase in serum amylase and lipase in pancreatitis was markedly lessened by a traditional Iranian drug, prepared from flower petals of *Echium amoenum*[33].

Mitochondrion is the organelle that generates most of the adenosine triphosphate (ATP) in mammalian cells. Oxidation of various substrates results in the formation of NADH or reduced ubiquinone, which then get oxidized through the electron transport chain of the mitochondria, to drive ATP synthesis. Generation of ATP is inevitably associated with production of ROS. ROS are highly reactive molecules, generated as metabolic by-products during ATP synthesis at major sites like complex-Ⅰ and complex-Ⅲ of electron transport chain.

Ethanol, when converted to acetaldehyde by ADH and to acetate by ALDH, a molecule of NADH is produced in each reaction, supplying more reducing equivalents (NADH) to mitochondria. These excess reducing equivalents facilitate transfer of electrons to molecular oxygen propagating the cycle of excess ROS generation. Shalbueva *et al* demonstrated that ethanol treatment led to a decrease in the NAD^+/NADH ratio in isolated acinar cells[34]. So ethanol increases redox pressure in mitochondria through NADH, promoting formation of ROS. The pathologic effect of cerulein in stimulating mitochondrial ROS production was reported to be by abnormal calcium signalling[6]. Once produced, ROS can cause potential damage to cellular constituents. Under physiological conditions, ROS are safely neutralized by the antioxidant defence systems both inside and outside the mitochondria.

In pancreatitis, infiltrating inflammatory cells, ethanol metabolism through CYP2E1, NADPH oxidase of PSCs and xanthine oxidase released by damaged pancreas could act as sources of intracellular ROS production[35-37]. Detoxifying enzymes (SOD, CAT, GPx) and non-enzymatic free radical scavengers (GSH) work together in cells against free radicals to preserve ideal redox status in living cells. When the ROS levels overcome the cellular antioxidant defence as in pancreatitis, the balance shifts towards ROS formation as noted in rats administered ethanol and cerulein. After treatment

Table 5. Effect of hydroalcoholic extract of licorice root (HAELR) on inflammatory markers.

Groups	MPO (Units/mg protein)	Caspase-1		IL-1 β (pg/mL)	IL-18 (pg/mL)
		Serum (pg/mL)	Pancreas (pM/mg protein)		
Control	2.93±0.33	12.30±1.76	12.50±1.41	14.90±1.65	190.30±30.03
HAELR	2.77±0.32	11.40±1.20	11.30±1.38	14.10±1.78	201.20±25.50
EtOH + Cerulein	5.04±0.69*	23.20±2.52*	48.80±5.27*	29.70±4.12*	345.50±42.10*
EtOH + Cerulein + HAELR	3.49±0.52#	15.10±1.89#	21.20±2.54#	19.30±2.10#	219.00±29.78#*

Data were analysed by one-way ANOVA followed by *post-hoc* Bonferroni test. Values are expressed as mean±SD of six rats in each group. MPO: myeloperoxidase; EtOH: ethanol. Statistical significance was calculated by comparing Control *vs.* EtOH + Cerulein; EtOH + Cerulein *vs.* EtOH + Cerulein + HAELR; $^{*}P=0.00$ and $^{\#}P<0.05$.

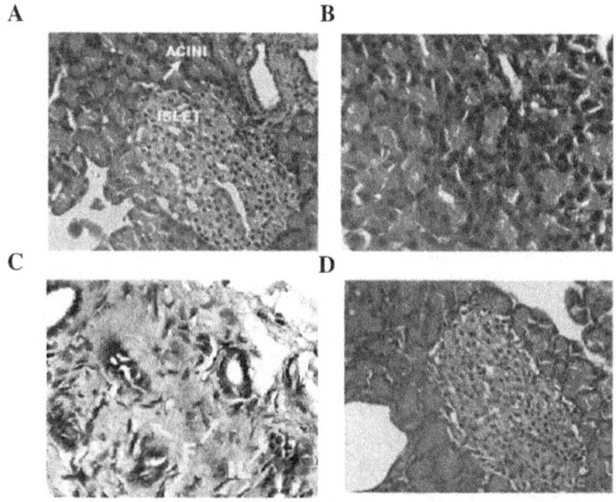

Figure 2. Histology of pancreatic tissue sections (H&E stain, 400×). (A)&(B) pancreas sections from the control rats and the rats treated with hydroalcoholic extract of licorice root alone show pristine tissue architecture; (C) sections from rats administered ethanol and cerulein show inflammatory cell infiltration (IL) and fibrosis (F); (D) sections from rats co-administered hydroalcoholic extract of licorice root show improved tissue architecture.

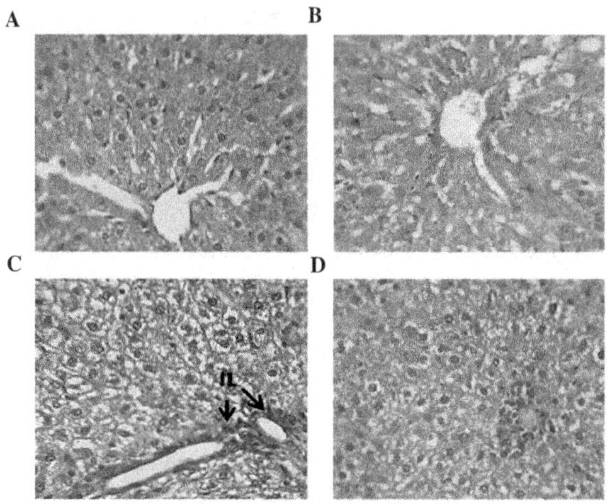

Figure 3. Histology of liver sections (H&E stain, 400×). (A)&(B) liver sections from the control rats and the rats treated with hydroalcoholic extract of licorice root alone show undisturbed structure; (C) liver tissues from rats administered ethanol and cerulein show inflammatory cell infiltration (IL); (D) liver sections from rats co-administered hydroalcoholic extract of licorice root show decreased infiltration of inflammatory cells.

with hydroalcoholic extract of licorice root, the enzyme levels were reverted towards normal, marking amelioration of oxidative stress.

Mitochondria, involved in the generation of ROS are the major targets of oxidative stress. Chronic ethanol treatment causes loss of mitochondrial GSH and inactivation of GPx and respiratory complexes. When these complexes are impaired, ROS can accumulate to toxic levels, leading to mitochondrial oxidative stress and dysfunction. Enhanced mitochondrial ROS production also induces NLRP3 inflammasome activation and associated inflammatory responses[38]. These aspects pertaining to mitochondria are focused separately in the other phase of our investigation.

Because of high chemical reactivity, ROS cause lipid peroxidation and the end products of lipid peroxidation like MDA and 4-HNE reflect the ROS-dependent tissue damage[39]. An increase in the levels of TBARS (MDA) and 4-HNE was observed in the pancreas of rats administered ethanol and cerulein, and these levels decreased significantly in rats co-administered hydroalcoholic extract of licorice root. These findings showed that treatment with hydroalcoholic extract of licorice root improved the antioxidant status and decreased the incidence of free radical-induced cell injury in pancreas.

Degree of polymorphonuclear leukocyte infiltration in the pancreas was measured in terms of tissue concentrations of MPO produced by these cells[40]. Elevation in MPO concentration was observed in the pancreas of rats received ethanol and cerulein, reflecting the tissue inflammation. MPO concentration decreased significantly in hydroalcoholic extract of licorice root treated rats, indicating its high anti-inflammatory potency. Bioactive compounds like flavonoids and saponins in hydroalcoholic extract of licorice root might contribute to its anti-inflammatory property.

ROS act as a molecular trigger of various inflammatory processes. A study by Yu *et al* has reported that cerulein generates ROS and thereby increases activation of NF-κB, and cytokine expression suggesting a possible relationship between ROS generation and the production of inflammatory cytokines in the pancreatic acinar cells. They further highlighted that these alterations are inhibited by endogenous antioxidants[41]. ROS can even act as a chemoattractant for inflammatory cells[6]. Caspase-1, IL-1β and IL-18 have important roles in mediating pancreatic injury and inflammation and their levels in serum significantly elevated after chronic ethanol exposure[42]. Persistent activation of PSCs by these cytokines propels pancreatic fibrosis. Existing studies revealed that, enhanced levels of IL-1β and IL-18 induce CP[43,44]. The serum levels of caspase-1, IL-1β and IL-18 in rats received ethanol and cerulein were higher compared to those of control rats, and decreased after hydroalcoholic extract of licorice root treatment, revealing its ability to inhibit the production of active IL-1β and IL-18. Similar inactivation was shown to reduce the severity of pancreatitis[45]. These observations draw special attention to highly potent anti-inflammatory nature of hydroalcoholic extract of licorice root. Histopathological observations showed that hydroalcoholic extract of licorice root co-administration ameliorated the pathological alterations in tissue architecture in both pancreas and liver, underlining its protective effect.

The results of this study clearly indicate that, hydroalcoholic extract of licorice root exhibits pancreato-protective activity probably by preventing the inflammatory cascade of cytokine activation and cellular injury. This anti-inflammatory effect of hydroalcoholic extract of licorice root as observed in this study might be due to its antioxidant phytoconstituents, since ethanol and cerulein-induced ROS production contributed to the severe inflammation in pancreas. Though many medicinal properties have been proved for licorice roots, this study confirms the anti-inflammatory property which protects pancreas from ethanol mediated injury.

Conflict of interest statement

The authors declare that they have no conflict of interest.

Acknowledgments

The authors thank the Sophisticated Analytical Instruments Facility, Indian Institute of Technology-Madras, Chennai, India, for providing the infrastructure and technical support for the GC-MS analysis.

References

[1] Manohar M, Verma AK, Venkateshaiah SU, Sanders NL, Mishra A. Pathogenic mechanisms of pancreatitis. *World J Gastrointest Pharmacol Ther* 2017; **8**(1): 10.

[2] Machicado JD, Yadav D. Epidemiology of recurrent acute and chronic pancreatitis: Similarities and differences. *Dig Dis Sci* 2017; **62**(7): 1683-1691.

[3] Deng X, Wang L, Elm MS, Gabazadeh D, Diorio GJ, Eagon PK, et al. Chronic alcohol consumption accelerates fibrosis in response to cerulein-induced pancreatitis in rats. *Am J Pathol* 2005; **166**(1): 93-106.

[4] Gukovskaya AS, Gukovsky I, Algül H, Habtezion A. Autophagy, inflammation, and immune dysfunction in the pathogenesis of pancreatitis. *Gastroenterology* 2017; **153**(5): 1212-1226.

[5] Apte MV, Pirola RC, Wilson JS. Alcohol and the pancreas. *Pancreapedia: Exocrine pancreas knowledge base*. American Pancreatic Association; 2016. Doi: 10.3998/panc.2016.17.

[6] Kim H. Cerulein pancreatitis: Oxidative stress, inflammation, and apoptosis. *Gut Liver* 2008; **2**(2): 74.

[7] Robles L, Vaziri ND, Ichii H. Role of oxidative stress in the pathogenesis of pancreatitis: Effect of antioxidant therapy. *Pancreat Disord Ther* 2013; **3**(1): 112.

[8] Mews P, Phillips P, Fahmy R, Korsten M, Pirola R, Wilson J, et al. Pancreatic stellate cells respond to inflammatory cytokines: Potential role in chronic pancreatitis. *Gut* 2002; **50**(4): 535-541.

[9] Gukovskaya AS, Hosseini S, Satoh A, Cheng JH, Nam KJ, Gukovsky I, et al. Ethanol differentially regulates NF-κB activation in pancreatic acinar cells through calcium and protein kinase C pathways. *Am J Physiol Gastrointest Liver Physiol* 2004; **286**(2): 204-213.

[10] Watanabe T, Kudo M, Strober W. Immunopathogenesis of pancreatitis. *Mucosal Immunol* 2017; **10**(2): 283.

[11] Xiang H, Zhang Q, Qi B, Tao X, Xia S, Song H, et al. Chinese herbal

medicines attenuate acute pancreatitis: Pharmacological activities and mechanisms. *Front Pharmacol* 2017; **8**: 216.

[12]Montero L, Ibáñez E, Russo M, di Sanzo R, Rastrelli L, Piccinelli AL, et al. Metabolite profiling of licorice (*Glycyrrhiza glabra*) from different locations using comprehensive two-dimensional liquid chromatography coupled to diode array and tandem mass spectrometry detection. *Anal Chim Acta* 2016; **913**: 145-159.

[13]Tewari D, Mocan A, Parvanov ED, Sah AN, Nabavi SM, Huminiecki L, et al. Ethnopharmacological approaches for therapy of jaundice: Part Ⅱ. Highly used plant species from Acanthaceae, Euphorbiaceae, Asteraceae, Combretaceae, and Fabaceae families. *Front Pharmacol* 2017; **8**: 519.

[14]Handa SS. An overview of extraction techniques for medicinal and aromatic plants. In: Handa SS, Khanuja SPS, Longo G, Rakesh DD (eds.) *Extraction technologies for medicinal and aromatic plants*. United nation industrial development organization and international center for Science and High Technology, Trieste, Italy; 2008, pp. 21-52.

[15]Hurst WJ, McKim JM, Martin Jr RA. High-performance liquid chromatographic determination of glycyrrhizin in licorice products. *J Agric Food Chem* 1983; **31**(2): 387-389.

[16]Lowry RR, Tinsley IJ. Rapid colorimetric determination of free fatty acids. *J Am Oil Chem Soc* 1976; **53**(7): 470-472.

[17]Gomori G. Assay of serum amylase with small amounts of serum. *Am J Clin Pathol* 1957; **27**: 714-715.

[18]Bradford MM. A rapid and sensitive method for the quantitation of microgram quantities of protein utilizing the principle of protein-dye binding. *Anal Biochem* 1976; **72**(1-2): 248-254.

[19]Moron MS, Depierre JW, Mannervik B. Levels of glutathione, glutathione reductase and glutathione S-transferase activities in rat lung and liver. *Biochim Biophys Acta* 1979; **582**(1): 67-78.

[20]Flohe L, Gunzler WA. Assays of glutathione peroxidase. *Methods Enzymol* 1984; **105**: 114-120

[21]Kakkar P, Das B, Viswanathan PN. A modified spectrophotometric assay of superoxide dismutase. *Indian J Biochem Biophys* 1984; **21**(2): 130-132.

[22]Aebi H. Catalase *in vitro*. *Methods Enzymol* 1984; **105**: 121-126

[23]Draper HH, Hadley M. Malondialdehyde determination as index of lipid peroxidation. *Methods Enzymol* 1990; **86**: 421-431.

[24]Bradley PP, Priebat DA, Christensen RD, Rothstein G. Measurement of cutaneous inflammation: Estimation of neutrophil content with an enzyme marker. *J Invest Dermatol* 1982; **78**(3): 206-209.

[25]Clemens DL, Schneider KJ, Arkfeld CK, Grode JR, Wells MA, Singh S. Alcoholic pancreatitis: New insights into the pathogenesis and treatment. *World J Gastrointest Pathophysiol* 2016; **7**(1): 48.

[26]Liu T, Zhang L, Joo D, Sun SC. NF-κB signaling in inflammation. *Signal Transduct Target Ther* 2017; **2**: 17023.

[27]Yu JY, Ha JY, Kim KM, Jung YS, Jung JC, Oh S. Anti-inflammatory activities of licorice extract and its active compounds, glycyrrhizic acid, liquiritin and liquiritigenin, in BV2 cells and mice liver. *Molecules* 2015; **20**(7): 13041-13054.

[28]Khattab HA, Abdel-Dayem UA, Jambi HA, Abbas AT, Abdul-Jawad MT, El-Shitany NA. Licorice (*Glycyrrhizza glabra*) extract prevents production of Th2 cytokines and free radicals induced by ova albumin in mice. *Int J Pharmacol* 2018; **14**(8): 1072-1079.

[29]Li YL, Guo H, Zhao YQ, Li AF, Ren YQ, Zhang JW. Quercetin protects neuronal cells from oxidative stress and cognitive degradation induced by amyloid β-peptide treatment. *Mol Med Rep* 2017; **16**(2): 1573-1577.

[30]Dhananjayan K. Molecular docking study characterization of rare flavonoids at the nac-binding site of the first bromodomain of BRD4 (BRD4 BD1). *J Cancer Res* 2015; **2015**: 1-15.

[31]Aljancić I, Stanković M, Tesević V, Vujisić L, Vajs V, Milosavljević S. Protective effect on human lymphocytes of some flavonoids isolated from two *Achillea* species. *Nat Prod Commun* 2010; **5**(5): 729-732.

[32]Wang XR, Hao HG, Chu L. Glycyrrhizin inhibits LPS-induced inflammatory mediator production in endometrial epithelial cells. *Microb Pathog* 2017; **109**: 110-113.

[33]Abed A, Minaiyan M, Ghannadi A, Mahzouni P, Babavalian MR. Effect of *Echium amoenum* Fisch. et Mey a traditional Iranian herbal remedy in an experimental model of acute pancreatitis. *ISRN Gastroenterol* 2012; **2012**: 141548

[34]Shalbueva N, Mareninova OA, Gerloff A, Yuan J, Waldron RT, Pandol SJ, et al. Effects of oxidative alcohol metabolism on the mitochondrial permeability transition pore and necrosis in a mouse model of alcoholic pancreatitis. *Gastroenterology* 2013; **144**(2): 437-446.

[35]Kikuta K, Masamune A, Satoh M, Suzuki N, Shimosegawa T. 4-hydroxy-2, 3-nonenal activates activator protein-1 and mitogen-activated protein kinases in rat pancreatic stellate cells. *World J Gastroenterol* 2004; **10**(16): 2344.

[36]Masamune A, Watanabe T, Kikuta K, Satoh K, Shimosegawa T. NADPH oxidase plays a crucial role in the activation of pancreatic stellate cells. *Am J Physiol Gastrointest Liver Physiol* 2008; **294**(1): G99-108.

[37]Folch E, Gelpi E, Rosello-Catafau J, Closa D. Free radicals generated by xanthine oxidase mediate pancreatitis-associated organ failure. *Dig Dis Sci* 1998; **43**(11): 2405-2410.

[38]Liu Q, Zhang D, Hu D, Zhou X, Zhou Y. The role of mitochondria in NLRP3 inflammasome activation. *Mol Immunol* 2018; **103**: 115-124.

[39]Kwiecien S, Jasnos K, Magierowski M, Sliwowski Z, Pajdo R, Brzozowski B, et al. Lipid peroxidation, reactive oxygen species and antioxidative factors in the pathogenesis of gastric mucosal lesions and mechanism of protection against oxidative stress-induced gastric injury. *J Physiol Pharmacol* 2014; **65**(5): 613-622.

[40]Simsek O, Kocael A, Kocael P, Orhan A, Cengiz M, Balcı H, et al. Inflammatory mediators in the diagnosis and treatment of acute pancreatitis: Pentraxin-3, procalcitonin and myeloperoxidase. *Arch Med Sci* 2018; **14**(2): 288.

[41]Yu JH, Lim JW, Namkung W, Kim H, Kim KH. Suppression of cerulein-induced cytokine expression by antioxidants in pancreatic acinar cells. *Lab Invest* 2002; **82**(10): 1359.

[42]Hoque R, Mehal WZ. Inflammasomes in pancreatic physiology and disease. *Am J Physiol Gastrointest Liver Physiol* 2015; **308**(8): G643-651.

[43]Marrache F, Tu SP, Bhagat G, Pendyala S, Österreicher CH, Gordon S, et al. Overexpression of interleukin-1β in the murine pancreas results in chronic pancreatitis. *Gastroenterology* 2008; **135**(4): 1277-1287.

[44]Schneider A, Haas SL, Hildenbrand R, Siegmund S, Reinhard I, Nakovics H, et al. Enhanced expression of interleukin-18 in serum and pancreas of patients with chronic pancreatitis. *World J Gastroenterol* 2006; **12**(40): 6507.

[45]Ning JW, Zhang Y, Yu MS, Gu ML, Xu J, Usman A, et al. Emodin alleviates intestinal mucosal injury in rats with severe acute pancreatitis *via* the caspase-1 inhibition. *Hepatobil Pancreat Dis Int* 2017; **16**(4): 431-436.

Journal of Applied Pharmaceutical Science Vol. 11(03), pp 130-140 March, 2021
Available online at http://www.japsonline.com
DOI: 10.7324/JAPS.2021.110316
ISSN 2231-3354

Glycyrrhizin modulates ER stress-induced UPR and concomitant mitochondrial dysfunction and activation of NF-κB in alcohol and cerulein-induced pancreatitis in rats

Sarmishta Srikantam[1], Geetha Arumugam[2*]
[1]Department of Biochemistry, Bharathi Womens College, Chennai, India.
[2]Principal, Dr. Ambedkar Government Arts College, Chennai, India.

ARTICLE INFO

Received on: 16/09/2020
Accepted on: 11/01/2021
Available online: 05/03/2021

Key words:
Pancreatitis, ER stress, mitochondrial oxidative stress, complex-1 impairment, calcium overload, glycyrrhizin.

ABSTRACT

Chronic pancreatitis (CP), a long-lasting pancreatic inflammatory illness, results predominantly from prolonged alcohol abuse. No standardized treatment exists so far. This investigation studies the effect of glycyrrhizin (GZ) on ethanol (EtOH) and cerulein (Cer)-induced pathology in the pancreas of male albino Wistar rats. Endoplasmic reticulum (ER) stress, mitochondrial damage, and activation of nuclear factor-κB (NF-κB) are the important pathomechanisms of CP. Rats were sorted as follows: Group 1 (control) and group 2 (GZ control) were given normal diet for the total period of 5 weeks, whereas group 3 (EtOH + Cer) and group 4 (EtOH +Cer+ GZ) were given alcoholic diet (0%–36%) for 4 weeks and Cer (20 μg/kg of body weight, IP) three times a week for the last 3 weeks to induce CP. Group 2 and group 4 rats were also given GZ (10 mg/kg of body weight, oral) from third week. GZ co-administration modulated ER stress by downregulating mRNA expression of unfolded protein response components like activating transcription factor 4, 78 kDa glucose-regulated protein (GRP78), CCAAT-enhancer-binding protein homologous protein (CHOP), X-box binding protein 1 and the inflammatory mediator, NF-κB. In addition, GZ ameliorated cellular oxidative stress. Measurements of calcium, complex-1 activity, and oxidative stress [including 4-hydroxynonenal (4-HNE)] in mitochondria substantiated the protective effect of GZ against mitochondrial dysfunction. Applying spearman's rank correlation (rs), a significant positive correlation between GRP78 versus 4-HNE ($p < 0.05$) and CHOP versus mitochondrial calcium ($p = 0.00$) was proved, which could indicate that ER stress and mitochondrial dysfunction act in concert to cause the pathobiology in CP. It can be concluded that GZ exhibits pancreato-protective effect against CP likely by targeting ER stress, NF-κB signaling, and by maintaining functional mitochondria.

INTRODUCTION

Chronic pancreatitis (CP) is a complex inflammatory disorder with progressive, irreversible deterioration, and fibrosis development in pancreas. Recurrent pancreatic injury caused by gallstone diseases (80%) and alcohol abuse (45%) leads to CP. Symptoms include disabling pain in the abdomen, pancreatic insufficiencies, malabsorption, and diabetes. CP can lead to pancreatic cancers (Uc *et al.*, 2016).

Pancreatic acinar cells of exocrine pancreas primarily produce and secrete digestive enzymes. Cholecystokinin is a gut hormone that regulates these enzyme secretions. However, supramaximal doses of cholecystokinin or its analog cerulein (Cer) cause injury to the pancreas, leading to pancreatitis. Ethanol (EtOH) weakens the recovery of injured pancreas. EtOH is metabolized in the pancreas and toxic metabolites like fatty acid ethyl esters (FAEEs), acetaldehyde, and byproducts like reactive oxygen species (ROS) are formed. Increased ROS production causes oxidative stress in the pancreas (Apte *et al.*, 1998). Cer induced pancreatitis is indicated by elevated levels of digestive enzymes and inflammatory cytokines in the serum (Deng *et al.*, 2005). An important mechanism initiating the entire inflammatory response is the up-regulation of genes encoding the secreted

*Corresponding Author
Geetha Arumugam, Dr. Ambedkar Government Arts College, Vyasarpadi, Chennai, India. E-mail: geethav21 @ yahoo.co.in

mediators like cytokines and chemokines. It takes place by the activation of nuclear factor-κB (NF-κB), a transcription regulator (Chen *et al.*, 2018).

Acinar cells have high rate of protein synthesis and so are typically abound in endoplasmic reticulum (ER). ER is involved in the assembly as well as folding of proteins. This function demands optimal redox conditions and calcium concentration. ER is a major intracellular calcium store. Various pathophysiological stimuli, like alcohol and ROS, through changes in calcium concentration lead to the build-up of abnormally folded proteins causing ER stress (Barrera *et al.*, 2018; Pandol *et al.*, 2010; Zeeshan *et al.*, 2016). A stress response called unfolded protein response (UPR) is initiated in the ER with the involvement of various stress sensing proteins like protein kinase RNA-like ER kinase (PERK), activating transcription factor 6 (ATF6), and inositol-requiring enzyme 1 (IRE1). Generally, these proteins are kept inactive by a 78 kDa glucose-regulated protein (GRP78). Their downstream signaling pathways include activating transcription factor 4 (ATF4), CCAAT-enhancer-binding protein homologous protein (CHOP), and X-box binding protein 1 (XBP1) which are aimed to restore homeostasis. However, if prolonged UPR and ER stress exist, homeostasis fails, leading to cytotoxic cellular damage (Cao and Kaufman, 2014; Chakrabarti *et al.*, 2011; Lugea *et al.*, 2015; Ye *et al.*, 2010).

Acinar cells are rich in mitochondria as secretion is energy-intensive. Among various organelles that interact with the ER, mitochondria are important. ER stress culminates in the release of calcium into the mitochondria (Marchi *et al.*, 2014). Mitochondrion is very sensitive to ensuing oscillatory increases in calcium levels and to ROS produced by alcohol metabolites (Trumbeckaite *et al.*, 2013).

Mitochondrial complex-1 is the prime component in the respiratory chain (ETC) of mitochondria. It transfers electrons from reduced nicotinamide adenine dinucleotide (NADH) to coenzyme Q leading to adenosine triphosphate (ATP) synthesis. Complex-1 is well recorded to be both an intracellular source and a target of ROS (Clemens *et al.*, 2014).

An ROS-generating mitochondrion can activate NLRP3 inflammasome, a multiprotein complex. NLRP3 can recognize damage associated molecular patterns generated by damaged mitochondria, serving as a signaling platform for the activation of caspase-1 and release of pro-inflammatory cytokines, interleukin-1β and interleukin-18. It is a key inflammasome involved in different inflammatory diseases, causing an inflammatory cell death. Mitochondria-induced NLRP3 inflammasome activation is implicated in inflammation (Gurung *et al.*, 2015; Zhou *et al.*, 2011).

Glycyrrhizin (GZ) (C42H62O16, 822.942 g/mol), a triterpene saponin, is a major constituent in licorice root (*Glycyrrhiza glabra*). GZ is widely used for treating peptic ulcers, hepatitis and to improve liver function. It is also used as anti-inflammatory, anti-oxidative, and immunomodulatory agent (Li *et al.*, 2014).

CP is an increasingly common disease lacking a specific targeted therapy. This study is intended to construct a multi-targeted treatment approach with the potent anti-oxidant, GZ, against EtOH and Cer-induced CP in rats. The focus being, mitigation of inflammation, oxidative stress and calcium overload in mitochondria, and ER stress amelioration.

MATERIALS AND METHODS

Chemicals

RNA later (Cat. #R0901) was procured from Sigma-Aldrich (Saint Louis, MO). GZ was obtained from Tokyo chemical industry chemicals (Chennai, India). Fura-2AM was from Merck (Mumbai, India). Alpha amylase and lipase kits were purchased from Coral Clinical Systems (Goa, India). Cer (product No.C9026-1MG) was from Sigma-Aldrich (Saint Louis, MO).

Experimental animals

Male albino Wistar rats (175–200 g) were housed in polyethylene cages on a 12 hours' light and dark cycle at a temperature of 25°C and humidity between 60% and 70%. Rats were given normal chow diet and water throughout acclimatization. The experimental design was reviewed and validated by the Institutional Animal Ethics Committee XIX/VELS/PCOL/06/2000/CPCSEA/IAEC/03.10.2016.

Induction of pancreatitis using EtOH and Cer

After a week of acclimatization, rats were grouped into four groups (six rats a group) as follows:

Group 1 (Control): normal chow diet and water *ad libitum* all through the 5-week study period (including acclimatization).

Group 2 (GZ control): normal chow diet and water *ad libitum* for 5 weeks and GZ at a dose of 10 mg/kg bodyweight, daily and orally for the last 3 weeks.

Group 3 (EtOH + Cer): isocaloric diet with ethanol (0%–36%) for 4 weeks and an IP injection of Cer (20 μg/kg body weight) three times per week for the last 3 weeks.

Group 4 (EtOH + Cer + GZ): isocaloric diet with ethanol (0%–36%) for 4 weeks, an IP injection of Cer (20 μg/kg body weight) three times per week for the last 3 weeks, along with the administration of GZ, at a daily oral dose of 10 mg/kg bodyweight, for the last 3 weeks.

After the study period, rats were fasted overnight, anesthetized using ether, and euthanized by cervical decapitation. Immediately blood was drawn, plasma and serum were separated and stored at 4°C until further analyses. Pancreas was excised and a portion of it was preserved in RNA later for quantitative polymerase chain reaction (qPCR) analysis.

Histopathological evaluation of pancreatitis

A portion of excised pancreas was cleansed with cold saline (0.9%) and then in formal saline (1:10) for 24 hours. The specimens were treated with alcohol, methyl benzoate and firmed up in paraffin wax. Tissue was then cut into 5 μm thickness and stained with hematoxylin and eosin for microscopic evaluation at 400× magnification.

Pancreatic mitochondrial isolation

Mitochondria was isolated from pancreatic tissue using mitochondria isolation kit for tissue (ab110168) obtained from Abcam (Cambridge, MA). Briefly, differential centrifugation of homogenized tissue samples was conducted (SPIN 1: 1,000 g 10 minutes 4°C for nuclei, SPIN 2: 12,000 g 15 minutes 4°C and repeatedly at 12,000 g for 15 minutes for mitochondria). Initially, the supernatant after first spin was segregated from nuclei and whole cells. It was then centrifuged again to achieve pellet rich in mitochondria. Concentration of protein in isolated mitochondria was quantified by Bradford protein assay (Bradford, 1976).

Biochemical Investigations

Determination of extent of pancreatic injury and cellular oxidative stress

Extent of pancreatic injury was monitored through activities of amylase and lipase using assay kits AMY(DS):01(P), LIP(UV):01(P), respectively. Besides, oxidative stress was measured through estimations of peroxide content and total antioxidant capacity (TAC). Their ratio oxidative stress index (OSI) was then calculated. The total peroxide content in plasma was estimated by ferrous oxidation-xylenol orange assay (Harma and Erel, 2003; Miyazawa, 1989). TAC was measured using 2,2'-azino-bis (3-ethyl benzothiazoline-6-sulfonic acid) method (Miller *et al*., 1993).

Assessment of neutrophil infiltration and other inflammatory mediators

Myeloperoxidase (MPO) was extracted from homogenized pancreas and its activity was assayed (Bradley *et al*., 1982). Serum levels of caspase-1 were estimated by an assay kit, ab39470 from Abcam, Cambridge, MA. Pro-inflammatory cytokines: interleukin-1β was assayed by an ELISA Kit, ab100767 from Abcam, Cambridge, MA, whereas interleukin-18 was estimated by an ELISA Kit, KRC2341 from Thermo Fisher scientific, Mumbai, India were determined.

Determination of mRNA expression of NF-κB and UPR components in ER stress by qPCR analysis

To perform qPCR, pancreas samples were initially processed for RNA isolation followed by conversion to cDNA. First, entire RNA was extracted by using trizol (Chomzynski and Mackey, 1995). RNA was then quantified using a spectrophotometer and the purity of the sample was determined using A260/280 readings. Samples were run on RNA gel to check for DNA contamination after being treated with DNase I from New England Biolabs (Catalogue#M0303S). RNA was converted to cDNA using cDNA reverse transcription kit from Thermo Fisher scientific, Mumbai, India (Catalogue#4368814). The qPCR analysis was performed using specific primer sequences (Table 1) synthesized at Eurofins genomics, Bangalore, India using Oligo perfect primer designer obtained from Thermo Fisher scientific, Mumbai, India. qPCR was performed on Stratagene Mx3000P PCR machine from Agilent technologies (Santa Clara, CA) using SYBR Green premix (Catalogue#RR420A) purchased from Takara Bio Inc, Japan. A two-step real time PCR with initial denaturation at 95°C for 10 minutes, followed by denaturation for about 30 seconds and annealing at 60°C for 60 seconds was performed. qPCR data was collected and analyzed on MxPro Software from Agilent technologies (Santa Clara, CA). Data was normalized using the comparative Ct values.

Table 1. Details of forward and reverse primers used in real-time PCR analysis.

Gene	Forward primer sequence	Reverse primer sequence
β-actin	5'-CACCAACTGGGACGACAT-3'	5'-ACAGCCTGGATAGCAACG-3'
ATF4	5'-TGAAAGAGAAGGCAGATT-3'	5'-TGAAAGAGAAGGCAGATT-3'
CHOP	5'-TGTTCTCTATTCGTTCCTAA-3'	5'-CCACCATCCTGAACTATT-3'
GRP78	5'-AATCAAGGTCTACGAAGG-3'	5'-AACACTGGTCCAACTAAG-3'
XBP1	5'-AACCTCTTAGATGACTTCCA-3'	5'-AGGCTGAACGATAACTGT-3'
NF-kB	5'-CAATCTTGATGTCATTCG-3'	5'-AAGTGTAATCCAATAGCA-3'

Determination of functional capacity of mitochondria

Determination of mitochondrial calcium $[Ca^{2+}]_m$

It was measured by changes in the intensity of fluorescence of mitochondrial isolates, loaded with a ratiometric calcium indicator, fura-2 AM. Mitochondrial isolates were dispersed in 0.25 M sucrose containing 1 mM EGTA and 20 mM Tris (pH 7.4). Then they were loaded with 10 μM fura-2 AM by incubating for 10 minutes at room temperature.

1 mg of fura-2 AM dissolved in 1 ml dimethyl sulfoxide was used as stock solution of fura-2 AM. For use, an aliquot of stock solution was diluted to 10 μM in modified Hanks' balanced salt solution (HBSS with Ca2+) immediately before loading. HBSS contains 137 mM of NaCl, 5.37 mM of KCl, 0.81 mM of $MgSO_4$, 0.44 mM of KH_2PO_4, 0.37 mM of Na_2HPO_4, 1.37 mM of $CaCl_2$, 5.56 mM of glucose (pH was adjusted to 7.2 with 10 mM 4-(2-hydroxyethyl)-1-piperazineethane sulfonic acid) (Lash and Jones, 1993). The mitochondrial suspensions were washed to remove excess fura-2 AM for measurement on a Jobin Yvon Fluorolog-3-11 spectrofluorometer with excitation wavelengths at 340 nm and 380 nm, emission wavelength at 510 nm as described before (Hotta *et al*., 2001; Trenker *et al*., 2008). Any change in the intramitochondrial free Ca2+ was measured as 340/380 ratio. The calcium concentrations from mitochondrial isolates of different experimental groups were calculated and expressed in nM by conversion of ratio values (Grynkiewicz *et al*., 1985).

Determination of mitochondrial dysfunction

Mitochondrial dysfunction was assessed by measuring its complex-1 activity using enzyme activity microplate assay kit (ab109721) obtained from Abcam (Cambridge, MA). This assay measures the NADH-dependent activity of complex-1 at OD 450 nm. The activity was expressed in terms of percentage activity of control, similar to that described previously for liver (Mukhopadhyay *et al*., 2014) and heart (Hao *et al*., 2015).

Determination of mitochondrial oxidative stress

Mitochondrial oxidative stress was assessed through estimations of reduced glutathione (GSH), glutathione peroxidase (GPx), superoxide dismutase (SOD), catalase (CAT), malondialdehyde (MDA), and 4-hydroxynonenal (4-HNE) levels. GSH level was determined according to Moron *et al*. (1979). Gpx was assayed as per Flohe and Gunzler. (Flohé and Günzler, 1984). Activity of SOD was estimated according to Kakkar *et al*. (1984). Activity of CAT was kinetically measured at 240 nm (Aebi, 1984).

Thiobarbituric acid-reactive substances (TBARS) assay was used to assess MDA production (Draper and Hadley, 1990). To measure 4-HNE, the mitochondrial fraction was allowed to react with dinitrophenylhydrazine (DNPH), mixed thoroughly and set aside for 1 hour, to derivatize 4-HNE in the sample. Then the formed adduct of 4-HNE and DNPH was extracted thrice with hexane and evaporated to dryness at 40°C. After cooling, 1 ml methanol was then added to all the samples and absorbance was measured at 350 nm using spectrophotometer (Kinter *et al*., 1994).

Statistical analysis of data

Statistical Package for the Social Sciences for Windows V.10 was used for the statistical calculations. The significance level was calculated by one-way analysis of variance (ANOVA) and post hoc Bonferroni. *P* values < 0.05 were reported significant. Spearman's correlation test was performed to identify the correlation between related data sets. The statistical significance (*p*-value) of correlation coefficient (r_s) was also determined.

RESULTS

Effect of GZ on altered histology of pancreas

Figure 1 depicts sections of pancreatic tissue (400×) from various study groups stained with hematoxylin and eosin. Pancreatic tissue from group 1 and group 2 rats showed no significant pathological manifestations of disease (Fig. 1A and B). In the sections of pancreatic tissue from EtOH and Cer given group 3 rats, a prominent infiltration by neutrophils indicating inflammation and mild fibrosis was observed (Fig. 1C). Pathological alterations caused by EtOH and Cer in the tissue architecture of pancreas were found to be ameliorated in GZ co-administered group 4 rats (Fig. 1D).

Effect of GZ on extent of pancreatic injury and cellular ROS

Amylase and lipase activities in serum were found elevated significantly upon administration of EtOH and Cer, compared to control. GZ co-administration found to have restored these levels significantly. These enzyme activities from all the four experimental groups were tabulated in Table 2 along with cellular oxidative stress and ROS through estimations of plasma total peroxide content, TAC and OSI.

Effect of GZ on neutrophil infiltration and release of inflammatory mediators

Pancreatic MPO activity and serum levels of inflammatory caspase-1, interleukin-1 β, and interleukin-18 in all study groups were shown in Table 3. Upon EtOH and Cer administration, levels of all these inflammatory mediators were found increased significantly compared to control. GZ co-administration was observed to reduce these levels significantly. There was no significant change in GZ control groups compared to control.

Effect of GZ on NF-κB expression

mRNA expressions of NF-κB in pancreatic tissues of various groups were shown in Figure 2. Upregulated expression

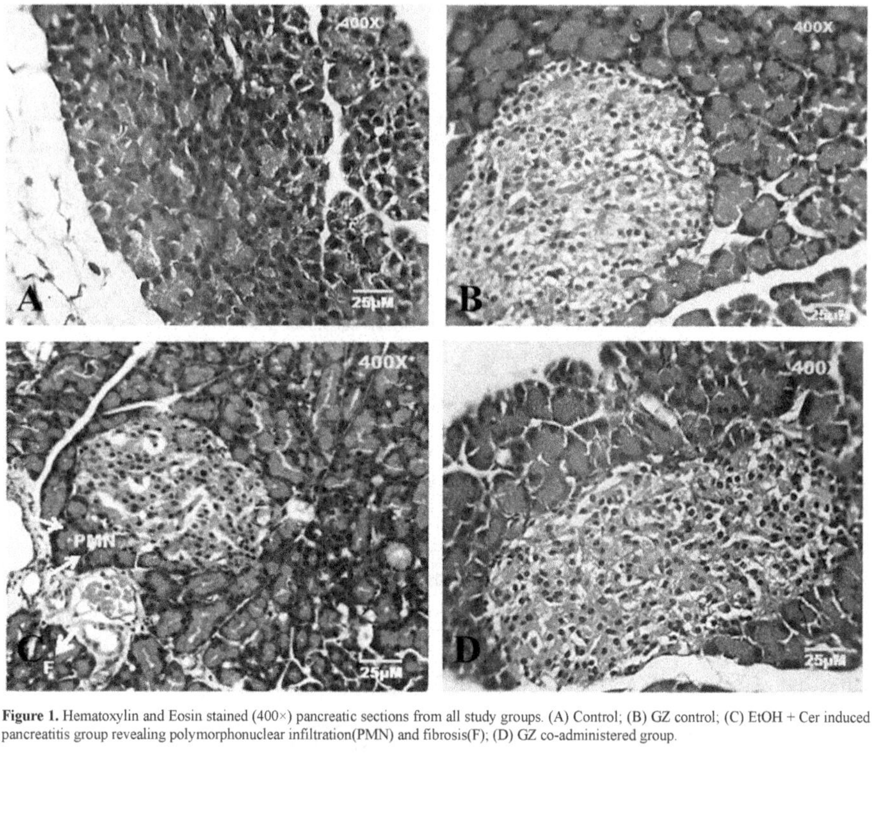

Figure 1. Hematoxylin and Eosin stained (400×) pancreatic sections from all study groups. (A) Control; (B) GZ control; (C) EtOH + Cer induced pancreatitis group revealing polymorphonuclear infiltration(PMN) and fibrosis(F); (D) GZ co-administered group.

Table 2. Effect of GZ treatment on enzyme markers of pancreatic injury and cellular ROS.

Group	Serum lipase (IU/l)	Serum amylase (IU/l)	Total peroxide (mmol/ml)	TAC (mmol trolox eq./l)	OSI
Control	149.1 ± 21.0	1662 ± 204.4	172.3 ± 20.8	332.4 ± 44.54	0.51 ± 0.05
GZ control	148.5 ± 18.0 NS	1607 ± 223.3 NS	169.8 ± 23.2NS	319.9 ± 45.10 NS	0.53 ± 0.06NS
EtOH + Cer	220.2 ± 28.6*	3118 ± 346*	287.5 ± 34.2*	227.1 ± 29.52*	1.26 ± 0.17*
EtOH + Cer + GZ	137.8 ± 16.6*	2297 ± 349.1*	194.0 ± 21.7*	302.5 ± 33.95*	0.64 ± 0.12*

Values represent mean ± S.D where n=6. Statistical significance was denoted through one-way ANOVA and post-hoc Bonferroni test by comparing control and GZ control; control and EtOH + Cer; EtOH + Cer and EtOH + Cer + GZ.
NS = not significant.
*p <0.05.

Table 3. Effect of GZ treatment on neutrophil infiltration and inflammation.

Groups	MPO (Units/mg protein)	Caspase-1 (pg/ml)	Interleukin-1β (pg/ml)	Interleukin-18 (pg/ml)
Control	2.1 ± 0.23	11.1 ± 1.60	13.75 ± 1.74	177.9 ± 20.4
GZ control	1.98 ± 0.25 NS	10.8 ± 1.54 NS	13.02 ± 1.62NS	169.1 ± 23.5NS
EtOH + Cer	3.7 ± 0.50*	96.4 ± 13.3*	29.6 ± 3.87*	302.5 ± 44.1*
EtOH + Cer + GZ	1.95 ± 0.29*	15.2 ± 2.06*	15.3 ± 1.79*	210.6 ± 31.5*

Values represent mean ± S.D where n = 6. Statistical significance was denoted through one-way ANOVA and post-hoc Bonferroni test by comparing control and GZ control; control and EtOH + Cer; EtOH + Cer and EtOH + Cer + GZ.
NS = not significant.
*p < 0.05.

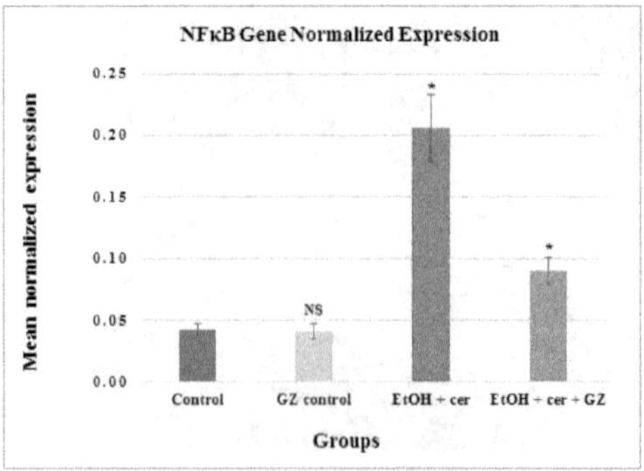

Figure 2. Gene expression analysis of NF-κB in pancreas studied by qPCR indicating the effect of GZ. y-axis represents mean normalized expression values expressed as mean ± S.D, where n = 6. Statistical significance was calculated through one-way ANOVA and post-hoc Bonferroni test by comparing control and GZ control; control and EtOH + Cer; EtOH + Cer and EtOH + Cer + GZ; *p < 0.05; NS = not significant.

of NF-κB was seen in EtOH and Cer given group 3 rats than in control. However, in GZ co-administered groups, the expression was found reduced significantly featuring its defense against persistent inflammation in CP.

Effect of GZ on mRNA expression of UPR components in ER stress

mRNA expression levels of UPR components like ATF4, GRP78, CHOP, XBP1 were provided in Figure 3a–d, respectively. In EtOH and Cer given rats, mRNA expression of these UPR genes was found upregulated significantly, indicating the chronically activated ER stress in CP. GZ co-administration was observed to ameliorate increased expression, underlining its protective effect against pathologic ER stress.

Effect of GZ on functional capacity of mitochondria

Effect of GZ on $[Ca^{2+}]_m$

Compared to control groups, the intra-mitochondrial free calcium was observed to be elevated significantly in group 3 rats (Table 4). This increase was not observed upon GZ co-administration, emphasizing attenuation of $[Ca^{2+}]_m$ overload by GZ. No significant change was observed in GZ control groups compared to control groups.

Effect of GZ on mitochondrial dysfunction

Complex-1 activities from mitochondrial isolates of various experimental groups were shown in Figure 4. Compared to control groups, pronounced decrease in complex-1 activity of mitochondrial ETC was observed in group 3 rats. It was observed to be restored upon GZ co-administration.

Effect of GZ on mitochondrial oxidative stress

A significant depletion in GSH content and antioxidant enzymes GPx, SOD, CAT was found in the mitochondrial fractions of group 3 rats than in control. Administration of GZ along with EtOH and Cer was recorded to enhance the antioxidative capacity of mitochondria (Table 4) as evidenced from attenuated levels. The lipid peroxidation levels, expressed in terms of TBARS and 4-HNE in mitochondrial fractions of EtOH and Cer given groups were found increased profoundly, compared to control (Table 4). Administration of GZ along with EtOH and Cer restored these levels, further highlighting its anti-oxidative nature.

Spearman's rank correlation analysis

Results of correlation analysis—GRP78 versus 4-HNE; CHOP versus IL-1 β, $[Ca^{2+}]_m$ and NF-κB; $[Ca^{2+}]_m$ versus TBARS,

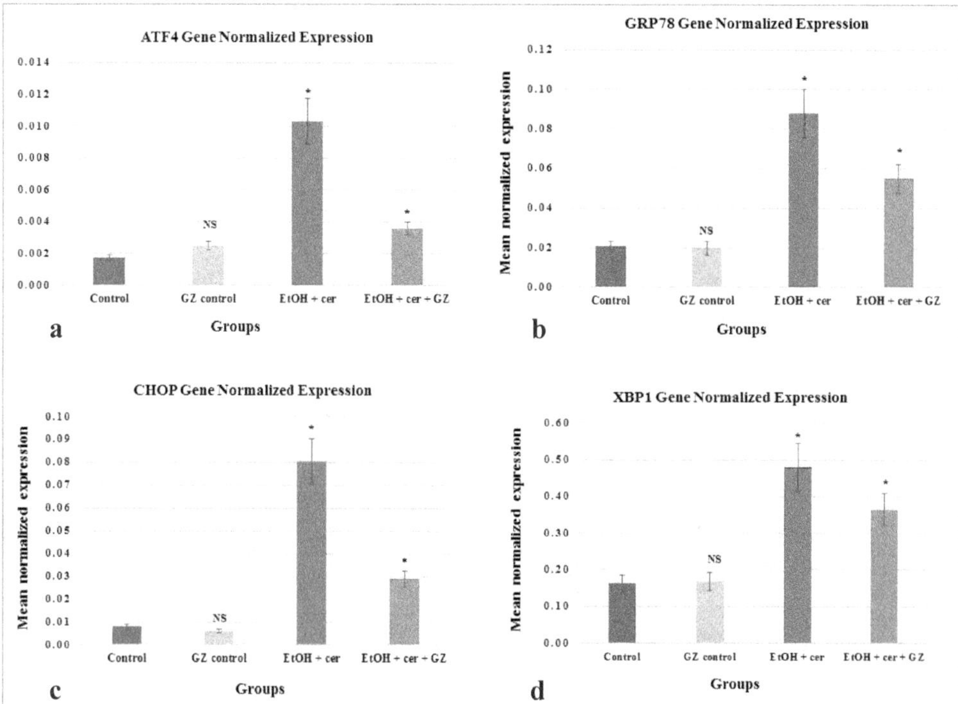

Figure 3. (a) Gene expression analysis of UPR components—ATF4 in pancreas, studied by qPCR indicating the effect of GZ. *y*-axis represents mean normalized expression values expressed as mean ± S.D, where $n = 6$. Statistical significance was calculated through one-way ANOVA and post-hoc Bonferroni test by comparing control and GZ control; control and EtOH + Cer; EtOH + Cer and EtOH + Cer + GZ; *$p < 0.05$; NS = not significant. (b) Gene expression analysis of UPR components—GRP78 in pancreas, studied by qPCR indicating the effect of GZ. *y*-axis represents mean normalized expression values expressed as mean ± S.D, where $n = 6$. Statistical significance was calculated through one-way ANOVA and post-hoc Bonferroni test by comparing control and GZ control; control and EtOH + Cer; EtOH + Cer and EtOH + Cer + GZ; *$p < 0.05$; NS = not significant. (c) Gene expression analysis of UPR components—CHOP in pancreas, studied by qPCR indicating the effect of GZ. *y*-axis represents mean normalized expression values expressed as mean ± S.D, where $n = 6$. Statistical significance was calculated through one-way ANOVA and post-hoc Bonferroni test by comparing control and GZ control; control and EtOH + Cer; EtOH + Cer and EtOH + Cer + GZ; *$p < 0.05$; NS = not significant. (d) Gene expression analysis of UPR components—XBP1 in pancreas, studied by qPCR indicating the effect of GZ. *y*-axis represents mean normalized expression values expressed as mean ± S.D, where $n = 6$. Statistical significance was calculated through one-way ANOVA and post-hoc Bonferroni test by comparing control and GZ control; control and EtOH + Cer; EtOH + Cer and EtOH + Cer + GZ; *$p < 0.05$; NS = not significant.

Table 4. Effect of GZ treatment on mitochondrial oxidative stress and $[Ca^{2+}]_m$.

Group	GSH (mg/g protein)	Gpx (nM GSH oxidized/minute/mg protein)	SOD (units/mg protein)	CAT (μ mol H_2O_2 consumed/minute/mg protein)	TBARS (nM/mg protein)	4-HNE (μM/g protein)	$[Ca^{2+}]_m$ (nM)
Control	4.8 ± 0.61	122.3 ± 16.38	6.9 ± 0.70	5.1 ± 0.57	8.6 ± 1.075	0.040 ± 0.006	91.63 ± 11.08
GZ control	4.6 ± 0.60^{NS}	119.7 ± 15.20^{NS}	6.7 ± 0.73^{NS}	4.8 ± 0.61^{NS}	9.2 ± 1.104^{NS}	0.035 ± 0.004^{NS}	93.7 ± 11.99^{NS}
EtOH +Cer	2.7 ± 0.39*	79.4 ± 11.43*	3.6 ± 0.42*	2.6 ± 0.26*	13.1 ± 1.89*	0.132 ± 0.017*	168.9 ± 20.09*
EtOH +Cer+ GZ	3.9 ± 0.43*	109.3 ± 14.20*	5.2 ± 0.62*	4.0 ± 0.48*	10.4 ± 1.16*	0.067 ± 0.007*	79.5 ± 9.14*

Values represent mean ± S.D where $n = 6$. Statistical significance was denoted through one-way ANOVA and post-hoc Bonferroni test by comparing control and GZ control; control and EtOH + Cer; EtOH + Cer and EtOH + Cer + GZ.
NS = not significant.
*$p < 0.05$.

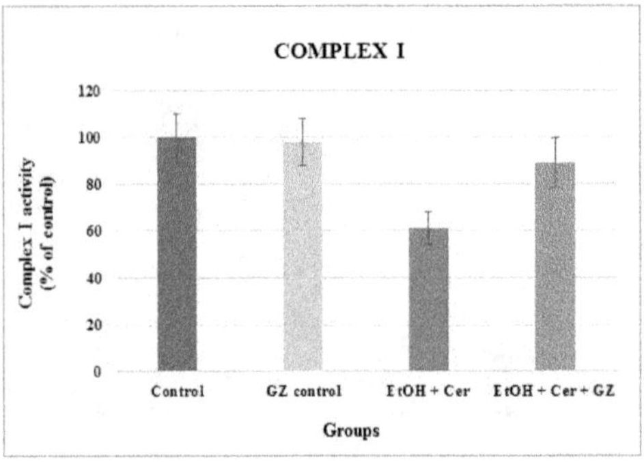

Figure 4. Complex-1 activity from mitochondrial isolates of various experimental groups indicating the attenuation of EtOH +Cer induced mitochondrial dysfunction by GZ. Values of GZ control, EtOH + Cer and EtOH + Cer + GZ were expressed as percentage activity of control.

Table 5. Spearman's rank correlation for different variables of study.

Parameter	r_s	*P*
GRP78 versus 4-HNE	0.78	<0.05
CHOP versus IL-1β	0.77	<0.05
CHOP versus $[Ca^{2+}]_m$	0.89	<0.001
CHOP versus NF-κB	0.81	<0.025
$[Ca^{2+}]_m$ versus complex-1	−0.82	<0.025
[Ca 2+]m versus TBARS	1.00	<0.001
$[Ca^{2+}]_m$ versus GSH	−0.71	0.05

r_s = spearman's correlation coefficient; P = statistical significance.

GSH and complex-1 were presented in Table 5. A strong negative correlation was seen between $[Ca^{2+}]_m$ and GSH; $[Ca^{2+}]_m$ and complex-1. And a strong positive correlation was observed among all the other data sets compared.

DISCUSSION

In the current study, protective effect of GZ against organelle dysfunction and chronic inflammation in CP was investigated in detail. These are the key pathological events for the progression of pancreatitis. No specific therapies for pancreatitis have been developed effectively so far except the supportive therapy (Frola *et al.*, 2019). CP was induced in rats by repeated dose of Cer combined with a sensitizing agent, EtOH. Cer hyperstimulation induces pancreatic injury in rats and EtOH aggravates this pathological effect towards CP, with clinical presentations like persistent inflammation (Deng *et al.*, 2005).

The functioning of pancreatic acinar cells depends on coordinated actions of ER and mitochondria. Previous studies clearly indicated that their functional ability has been disturbed in pancreatitis (Gukovskaya *et al.*, 2016). Physiologically, pancreatic digestive enzymes are synthesized in ER of pancreatic acini, transported as inactive pro-enzymes and get activated only in the small intestine. Accurate protein processing by ER is extremely important, to avoid any premature activation of pancreatic enzymes in acinar cells itself. Cytosolic calcium concentration and calcium release from intracellular calcium pools (primarily ER), in response to hormonal stimuli is a signaling mechanism for this process. Metabolites of EtOH like FAEE and other fatty acids, along with Cer were shown to induce gradual release of calcium from ER (called calcium store depletion) leading to pathological calcium signaling patterns (Criddle *et al.*, 2006). It can induce premature activation of pancreatic enzymes and pancreatic tissue destruction. Thus, injured pancreatic acini facilitate the release of pancreatic enzymes into the blood stream. The enzyme markers of EtOH and Cer-induced pancreatic injury are lipase and amylase activities, which are generally monitored in serum (Frulloni *et al.*, 2005). In this investigation, increased serum levels of these enzymes were found in EtOH and Cer-given group 3 rats and these serological alterations were found to be ameliorated with GZ co-administration.

ER, an important organelle for protein folding and calcium storage; mitochondria, which interpret intracellular calcium signals by taking up and releasing calcium are the two key cellular organelles most disordered in EtOH and Cer-induced injury (Lugea *et al.*, 2015). Administration of EtOH can perturb ER homeostasis, by imparting aggregation of improperly folded nascent polypeptides, causing substantial activation of UPR and ER stress. Acinar cells may be prompted to injury and death in due course (Criddle *et al.*, 2007). Oxidative stress could be a probable mechanism behind the induction of pancreatic ER stress by EtOH. A study by Waldron *et al.* (2018) has shown that EtOH through its oxidative effect caused deformities in the structure of ER, promoting ER stress-related pathology in mouse pancreas. And all these pathological changes are further aggravated in response to Cer. Chronic ER stress is well recorded to be a primary cellular pathomechanism of pancreatitis.

In this study, ER stress was studied by monitoring the mRNA expressions of its UPR components—GRP78, ATF4, CHOP, XBP1. ATF4 is involved in the transcription of genes needed to rebuild ER homeostasis and activates the genes encoding antioxidative stress responses. ATF4 also activates genes responsible for the regulation of intracellular redox status and GSH synthesis. CHOP/GADD153, a transcription factor of ER stress is a 29 kDa protein which is required in apoptosis promoted by ER stress (Lugea *et al.*, 2015). Elevated CHOP is related to uncontrolled inflammation as it regulates cytokine production and promotes increased number of inflammatory cells. CHOP also causes the production of interleukin-1 β by triggering caspase-1 through caspase-11, leading to inflammatory stress responses (Nishitoh, 2012). Protein processing in ER is executed by various chaperones. GRP78 is an abundant ER-specific chaperone belonging to HSP70 family and this protein inactivates other chaperones like PERK, IRE1, and ATF6, which relate ER stress to UPR stimulation. When unfolded proteins pile up, GRP78 leaves the three receptors leading to the stimulation of these receptors and triggering of respective UPR pathways. GRP78 is very sensitive to ER stress (Chaudhari *et al.*, 2014). XBP1 is an active factor of transcription for the production of GRP78. Overexpression of mRNA level of XBP1 was documented previously in CP. Stimulation of IRE1/XBP1 pathway is a cellular stress response to reinstate protein processing in ER (Sah *et al.*, 2014). Together, the UPR mechanisms alleviate ER stress to maintain ER homeostasis. It is very important for a functional acinar cell during both normal and diseased states. But if the ER stress is not rectified, persistent stimulation of the UPR takes place.

In the study, a sustained up-regulation of mRNA expressions of all the four UPR components—ATF4, CHOP, GRP78, and XBP1 was seen in EtOH and Cer-given group, which revealed the existence of persistent ER stress. GZ co-administration significantly reduced the EtOH and Cer-induced ER stress as observed from downregulated expression of these genes in GZ co-administered rats. Lugea *et al.* (2015) hypothesized that pancreas initiates this adaptive UPR to reduce the ER stress generated by alcohol. But when it is beyond the protective capacity of UPR, it progresses to CP. Our study highlighted the pancreas-protective effect of GZ in EtOH and Cer-induced CP with UPR as a definitive target.

Generally, acinar cells contain high number of mitochondria as energy source for the synthesis of digestive enzymes. Pancreatic mitochondria are more susceptible intracellular targets to EtOH-induced injury. Both non-oxidative and oxidative metabolism of alcohol disturbs pancreatic mitochondrial functions and causes acinar cell death by aberrant calcium signaling (Clemens *et al.*, 2014). As the excess calcium released from ER, in response to alcoholic metabolites is received by pancreatic mitochondria, sustained elevation of mitochondrial calcium takes place. Mitochondria depict the primary intracellular origin for the production of ROS. Physiologically, many superoxides and hydrogen peroxides are formed during mitochondrial ETC. Mitochondrial ROS further promotes calcium release from nearby ER and increases $[Ca^{2+}]_m$ accumulation, initiating a positive feedback cycle. Excessive flow of calcium to mitochondria leads to calcium stimulated oxidative damage to mitochondria, failure of ATP production, energy deprivation, and cellular necrosis (Cao and Kaufman, 2014). Toxic accumulation of ROS is usually countered by GSH, SOD, and CAT. To investigate the mitochondrial oxidative stress, GSH, GPx, SOD, and CAT were monitored. Oxidative stress disrupts mitochondrial membrane, as shown by excess lipid peroxidation products like TBARS and 4-HNE, affecting permeability. A significant decrease in the levels of antioxidants accompanied by an increase in lipid peroxidation products was noticed in EtOH and Cer-given group 3 rats than in control. Co-administering GZ restrained these changes. Reduced enzyme activities of SOD and GPx lead to oxidative stress in mitochondria (Zang *et al.*, 2007). Alteration in the mitochondrial function is one of the mechanisms for the onset and progression of pancreatitis. It has been observed that, GZ treatment can be a good strategy to target mitochondria, in order to locally scavenge ROS at their site of origin itself. mitoquinone and 10-(6'-plastoquinonyl) decyltriphenylphosphonium are the other mitochondria targeted antioxidants proved to be effective against pancreatitis, by acting as scavengers of ROS (Huang *et al.*, 2015; Weniger *et al.*, 2016).

ER stress and mitochondrial oxidative stress are interlinked phenomena regulated through calcium. Calcium serves as a second messenger for many cellular processes. To determine the $[Ca^{2+}]_m$ concentration, fura-2AM which is a membrane permeable, non-invasive, ratiometric indicator was used. It can accumulate to a variable extent when loaded onto mitochondrial isolates (Sheu and Sharma, 1999). Excitation wavelengths used to determine Bound-Ca^{2+} fura-2 AM and free-Ca^{2+} fura-2 AM are 340 nm and 380 nm, respectively. Fura-2 AM emits at 510 nm for both the states. The ratio of 510 nm to 340 nm and 510 nm to 380 nm indicates the calcium levels (Grynkiewicz *et al.*, 1985). In the study, $[Ca^{2+}]_m$ concentration in EtOH and Cer-given group 3 rats was found increased significantly than in control and GZ co-administered group 4 rats. Although modest increase in $[Ca^{2+}]_m$ concentrations enhances enzymatic activity and subsequent ATP synthesis, excessive $[Ca^{2+}]_m$ load may disable ATP synthetic pathways (Brookes *et al.*, 2004). The results showed attenuation of $[Ca^{2+}]_m$ overload by GZ. Odinokova *et al.* (2009) suggested that both the ROS and calcium in mitochondria regulate the functional status of acinar cells during pancreatitis and further highlighted that stabilizing mitochondria against such functional loss may be a good approach to reduce the severity of pancreatitis. Mitochondrial cytochrome C is released under the influence of $[Ca^{2+}]_m$ overload and excess ROS. The loss of cytochrome C has been shown to inhibit the ETC leading to mitochondrial dysfunction.

Mitochondrial dysfunction was assessed through complex-1 activity in the isolated mitochondria. Complex-1 is the gate keeper of ETC and is reported to be severely affected in oxidative stress (Wu *et al.*, 2015). Early organ specific pancreatic mitochondrial dysfunction in Cer-induced pancreatitis was described by various studies (Trumbeckaite *et al.*, 2013). EtOH affects the mitochondrial functioning through its oxidative metabolite acetaldehyde, which destabilizes the ETC (Manzo-Avalos and Saavedra-Molina, 2010). In this study, marked inhibition of mitochondrial complex-1 activity was observed upon EtOH and Cer administration and it was found to be restored with GZ co-administration. Mitochondrial compex-1 is positioned in the inner membrane of mitochondria, which is prone to lipid peroxidation. The formed 4-HNE can produce HNE-protein adducts with complex-1, affecting its function. It was illustrated in mitochondrial isolates of diabetic rat kidney by Wu *et al.* (2015). Sun *et al.* (2016) demonstrated that chronic alcohol feeding to rats increases the 4-HNE levels in liver mitochondria leading to impaired functioning of respiratory complexes. The defective complexes of ETC can further exacerbate ROS generation in mitochondria. GZ co-administration prevented the loss in activity of complex-1 and this might be by modulating 4-HNE level, underlining its protection against mitochondrial damage in CP.

Sustained ER stress activates inflammatory pathways through chronic NF-κB activation in CP (Sah *et al.*, 2014). We observed an up-regulated mRNA expression of NF-κB in EtOH and Cer-given group and, GZ co-administration was found to counteract it. NF-κB is held ineffective by IκBα, an inhibitor of NF-κB in normal cells. Many studies have shown ER stress to downregulate IκBα leading to NF-κB activation. EtOH also causes activation of NF-κB directly through the activation of protein kinase C in pancreatic acini (Gukovskaya *et al.*, 2004). NF-κB integrates ER stress with pro-inflammatory response through a protein called tumor necrosis factor α receptor-associated factor2 that activates NF-kB, promoting its nuclear translocation. The activated NF-κB promotes expression of pro-inflammatory cytokines and chemokines increasing the severity of pancreatitis. It has also been well documented that, inhibition of NF-κB improves pancreatic function (Huang *et al.*, 2013).

Correlation analysis is a statistical method to find out the strength of a relationship between two sets of data. The Spearman's rank correlation was measured between GRP78 versus 4-HNE; CHOP versus IL-1β, $[Ca^{2+}]_m$; $[Ca^{2+}]_m$ versus complex-1,

TBARS and GSH; CHOP versus NF-κB. Rs value, and its statistical significance level based on exact critical probability (p) values were calculated. Considering the small p values, the null hypothesis was rejected and the relationship between compared datasets was found significant. In the study, a positive correlation was noticed between GRP78 versus 4-HNE and CHOP versus IL-1β, $[Ca^{2+}]_m$. A correlated effect was observed between ER stress and mitochondrial dysfunction, the key mechanisms contributing to the pathobiology of CP.

Moreover, histological observations in the study evidenced a prominent neutrophil infiltration and mild fibrosis in pancreatic sections of EtOH and Cer-given groups which is a characteristic feature of CP. This was found to be counteracted by GZ, as observed in pancreatic sections of GZ co-administered rats. The reason behind this excessive inflammatory response in group 3 rats is perhaps the NF-κB activation, as noted in this study. The transcription of NF-κB genes is often activated by cellular ROS (Morgan and Liu, 2011). The attenuation of NF-κB activation by GZ in our study is probably by influencing the cellular ROS levels as shown by total peroxide content, TAC and OSI levels. In a similar study, Morin which is an anti-inflammatory flavone has been found to reduce activation of NF-κB by its anti-oxidant properties (Kim *et al*., 2010).

ER stress-induced mitochondrial damage and associated ROS also cause activation of NLRP3 inflammasome and associated inflammatory responses that worsen pancreatitis. Mitochondrial ROS was shown to activate NLRP3 inflammasome directly. NLRP3 inflammasome is assembled from its component proteins, namely, NLRP3 sensor, apoptosis-associated speck-like protein containing a caspase activation and recruitment domain and caspase-1. Upon activation, caspase-1 cleaves pro-interleukin1β and pro-interleukin 18 into inflammatory cytokines interleukin-1β and interleukin-18 that mediates pancreatic tissue injury (Liu *et al*., 2018). In the present investigation, the serum levels of caspase-1, interleukin-1β, and interleukin-18 were noticed to be increased in EtOH and Cer-given rats and GZ co-administration observed to counteract these modifications, highlighting its ability to reduce the disease severity. The energy deficits with mitochondrial complex-1 impairment and mitochondrial oxidative stress, accompanied by excessive unfolded ER proteins impair ER-mitochondrial cooperation, promoting inflammatory responses. The basic therapy for CP is the treatment of pain and underlying inflammation. Many anti-inflammatory agents like thalidomide, panhematin, montelukast, dantrolene were documented to be effective against pancreatitis (Sah and Saluja, 2011).

CONCLUSION

From the study, it could be conjectured that GZ ameliorates the pancreatic impairment in CP by targeting the UPR, NF-κB mediated NLRP3 inflammasome activation, and cytokine maturation, in addition to preserving the functional ability of the mitochondria. GZ is observed to influence the heat shock protein GRP78. Its potential to influence other molecular chaperones like HSP27, HSP60, HSP70, and HSP90 known to be involved in pancreatic pathophysiology, could hold a valuable therapeutic potential. An *in silico* docking study could be performed to compute the ability of GZ to interact with UPR, NLRP3 component proteins and heat shock proteins, to further confirm the drug-like property of GZ.

AUTHOR CONTRIBUTIONS

All authors made substantial contributions to conception and design, acquisition of data, or analysis and interpretation of data; took part in drafting the article or revising it critically for important intellectual content; agreed to submit to the current journal; gave final approval of the version to be published; and agree to be accountable for all aspects of the work. All the authors are eligible to be an author as per the international committee of medical journal editors (ICMJE) requirements/guidelines.

FUNDING

There is no funding to report.

CONFLICTS OF INTEREST

The authors report no financial or any other conflicts of interest in this work.

PUBLISHER'S NOTE

This journal remains neutral with regard to jurisdictional claims in published institutional affiliation.

REFERENCES

Aebi H. Catalase *in vitro*. Methods Enzymol, 1984; 105:121–6.

Apte MV, Haber PS, Norton ID, Wilson JS. Alcohol and the pancreas. Addict Biol, 1998; 3(2):137–50.

Barrera K, Stanek A, Okochi K, Niewiadomska Z, Mueller C, Ou P, John D, Alfonso AE, Tenner S, Huan C. Acinar cell injury induced by inadequate unfolded protein response in acute pancreatitis. World J Gastrointest Pathophysiol, 2018; 9(2):37.

Bradford MM. A rapid and sensitive method for the quantitation of microgram quantities of protein utilizing the principle of protein-dye binding. Anal Biochem, 1976; 72(1–2):248–54.

Bradley PP, Priebat DA, Christensen RD, Rothstein G. Measurement of cutaneous inflammation: estimation of neutrophil content with an enzyme marker. J Invest Dermatol, 1982; 78(3):206–9.

Brookes PS, Yoon Y, Robotham JL, Anders MW, Sheu SS. Calcium, ATP, and ROS: a mitochondrial love-hate triangle. Am J Physiol Cell Physiol, 2004; 287(4):C817–33.

Cao SS, Kaufman RJ. Endoplasmic reticulum stress and oxidative stress in cell fate decision and human disease. Antioxid Redox Signal, 2014; 21(3):396–413.

Chakrabarti A, Chen AW, Varner JD. A review of the mammalian unfolded protein response. Biotechnol Bioeng, 2011; 108(12):2777–93.

Chaudhari N, Talwar P, Parimisetty A, Lefebvre d'Hellencourt C, Ravanan P. A molecular web: endoplasmic reticulum stress, inflammation, and oxidative stress. Front Cell Neurosci, 2014; 8:213.

Chen L, Deng H, Cui H, Fang J, Zuo Z, Deng J, Li Y, Wang X, Zhao L. Inflammatory responses and inflammation-associated diseases in organs. Oncotarget, 2018; 9(6):7204.

Chomzynski P, Mackey K. Modification of the TRI reagent [TM] procedure for isolation of RNA from polysaccharide-and proteoglycan-rich sources. Biotechniques, 1995; 19:942–5.

Clemens DL, Wells MA, Schneider KJ, Singh S. Molecular mechanisms of alcohol associated pancreatitis. World J Gastrointest Pathophysiol, 2014; 5(3):147.

Criddle DN, Gerasimenko JV, Baumgartner HK, Jaffar M, Voronina S, Sutton R, Petersen OH, Gerasimenko OV. Calcium signalling and pancreatic cell death: apoptosis or necrosis? Cell Death Differ, 2007; 14(7):1285–94.

Criddle DN, Murphy J, Fistetto G, Barrow S, Tepikin AV, Neoptolemos JP, Sutton R, Petersen OH. Fatty acid ethyl esters cause pancreatic calcium toxicity via inositol trisphosphate receptors and loss of ATP synthesis. Gastroenterology, 2006; 130(3):781–93.

Deng X, Wang L, Elm MS, Gabazadeh D, Diorio GJ, Eagon PK, Whitcomb DC. Chronic alcohol consumption accelerates fibrosis in response to cerulein-induced pancreatitis in rats. Am J Pathol, 2005; 166(1):93–106.

Draper HH, Hadley M. Malondialdehyde determination as index of lipid Peroxidation. Methods Enzymol, 1990; 186:421–31.

Flohé L, Günzler WA. Assays of glutathione peroxidase. Methods Enzymol, 1984; 105:114–20.

Frola C, Somasundaram M, Hariharan D, Kolaityte V, Mohandas S, Stättner S, Yip VS. The role of surgery in chronic pancreatitis. Eur Surg, 2019; 51(3):114–20.

Frulloni L, Patrizi F, Bernardoni L, Cavallini G. Pancreatic hyperenzymemia: clinical significance and diagnostic approach. JOP, 2005; 6(6):536–51.

Grynkiewicz G, Poenie M, Tsien RY. A new generation of Ca2+ indicators with greatly improved fluorescence properties. J Biol Chem, 1985; 260(6):3440–50.

Gukovskaya AS, Hosseini S, Satoh A, Cheng JH, Nam KJ, Gukovsky I, Pandol SJ. Ethanol differentially regulates NF-κB activation in pancreatic acinar cells through calcium and protein kinase C pathways. Am J Physiol Gastrointest Liver Physiol, 2004; 286(2):G204–13.

Gukovskaya AS, Pandol SJ, Gukovsky I. New insights into the pathways initiating and driving pancreatitis. Curr Opin Gastroenterol, 2016; 32(5):429–435

Gurung P, Lukens JR, Kanneganti TD. Mitochondria: diversity in the regulation of the NLRP3 inflammasome. Trends Mol Med, 2015; 21(3):193–201.

Hao E, Mukhopadhyay P, Cao Z, Erdélyi K, Holovac E, Liaudet L, Lee WS, Haskó G, Mechoulam R, Pacher P. Cannabidiol protects against doxorubicin-induced cardiomyopathy by modulating mitochondrial function and biogenesis. Mol Med, 2015; 21(1):38–45.

Harma M, Erel O. Increased oxidative stress in patients with hydatidiform mole. Swiss Med Wkly, 2003; 133(4142):563–6.

Hotta Y, Ishikawa N, Ohashi N, Matsui K. Effects of SM-20550, a selective Na+-H+ exchange inhibitor, on the ion transport of myocardial mitochondria. Mol Cell Biochem, 2001; 219(1–2):83–90.

Huang H, Liu Y, Daniluk J, Gaiser S, Chu J, Wang H, Li ZS, Logsdon CD, Ji B. Activation of nuclear factor-κB in acinar cells increases the severity of pancreatitis in mice. Gastroenterology, 2013; 144(1):202–10.

Huang W, Cash N, Wen L, Szatmary P, Mukherjee R, Armstrong J, Chvanov M, Tepikin AV, Murphy MP, Sutton R, Criddle DN. Effects of the mitochondria-targeted antioxidant mitoquinone in murine acute pancreatitis. Mediators Inflamm, 2015; 2015:901780

Kakkar P, Das B, Viswanathan PN. A modified spectrophotometric assay of superoxide dismutase. Indian J Biochem Biophys, 1984; 21(2):130–2.

Kim JM, Lee EK, Park G, Kim MK, Yokozawa T, Yu BP, Chung HY. Morin modulates the oxidative stress-induced NF-κB pathway through its anti-oxidant activity. Free Radic Res, 2010; 44(4):454–61.

Kinter M, Robinson CS, Grimminger LC, Gillies PJ, Shimshick EJ, Ayers C. Whole blood and plasma concentrations of 4-hydroxy-2-nonenal in Watanabe heritable hyperlipidemic versus New Zealand White rabbits. Biochem Biophys Res Commun, 1994; 199(2):671–5.

Lash LH, Jones DP. Mitochondrial dysfunction: methods in toxicology. Elsevier, Amsterdam, Netherlands, 1993.

Li JY, Cao HY, Liu P, Cheng GH, Sun MY. Glycyrrhizic acid in the treatment of liver diseases: literature review. Biomed Res Int, 2014; 2014:872139.

Liu Q, Zhang D, Hu D, Zhou X, Zhou Y. The role of mitochondria in NLRP3 inflammasome activation. Mol immunol, 2018; 103:115–24.

Lugea A, Waldron RT, Pandol SJ. Pancreatic adaptive responses in alcohol abuse: role of the unfolded protein response. Pancreatology, 2015; 15(4): S1–5.

Manzo-Avalos S, Saavedra-Molina A. Cellular and mitochondrial effects of alcohol consumption. Int J Environ Res Public Health, 2010; 7(12):4281–304.

Marchi S, Patergnani S, Pinton P. The endoplasmic reticulum–mitochondria connection: one touch, multiple functions. Biochim Biophys Acta, 2014; 1837(4):461–9.

Miller NJ, Rice-Evans C, Davies MJ, Gopinathan V, Milner A. A novel method for measuring antioxidant capacity and its application to monitoring the antioxidant status in premature neonates. Clin Sci, 1993; 84(4):407–12.

Miyazawa T. Determination of phospholipid hydroperoxides in human blood plasma by a chemiluminescence-HPLC assay. Free Radic Biol Med, 1989; 7(2):209–18.

Morgan MJ, Liu ZG. Crosstalk of reactive oxygen species and NF-κB signaling. Cell Res, 2011; 21(1):103–15.

Moron MS, Depierre JW, Mannervik B. Levels of glutathione, glutathione reductase and glutathione S-transferase activities in rat lung and liver. Biochim Biophys Acta, 1979; 582(1):67–78.

Mukhopadhyay P, Rajesh M, Cao Z, Horváth B, Park O, Wang H, Erdelyi K, Holovac E, Wang Y, Liaudet L, Hamdaoui N. Poly (ADP-ribose) polymerase-1 is a key mediator of liver inflammation and fibrosis. Hepatology, 2014; 59(5):1998–2009.

Nishitoh H. CHOP is a multifunctional transcription factor in the ER stress response. J Biochem, 2012; 151(3):217–9.

Odinokova IV, Sung KF, Mareninova OA, Hermann K, Evtodienko Y, Andreyev A, Gukovsky I, Gukovskaya AS. Mechanisms regulating cytochrome c release in pancreatic mitochondria. Gut, 2009; 58(3):431–42.

Pandol SJ, Gorelick FS, Gerloff A, Lugea A. Alcohol abuse, endoplasmic reticulum stress and pancreatitis. Dig Dis, 2010; 28(6):776–82.

Sah RP, Garg SK, Dixit AK, Dudeja V, Dawra RK, Saluja AK. Endoplasmic reticulum stress is chronically activated in chronic pancreatitis. J Biol Chem, 2014; 289(40):27551–61.

Sah RP, Saluja A. Molecular mechanisms of pancreatic injury. Curr Opin Gastroenterol, 2011; 27(5):444.

Sheu SS, Sharma VK. A novel technique for quantitative measurement of free Ca2+ concentration in rat heart mitochondria. J Physiol, 1999; 518(2):577–84.

Sun Q, Zhong W, Zhang W, Zhou Z. Defect of mitochondrial respiratory chain is a mechanism of ROS overproduction in a rat model of alcoholic liver disease: role of zinc deficiency. Am J Physiol Gastrointest Liver Physiol, 2016; 310(3):G205–14.

Trenker M, Fertschai I, Malli R, Graier WF. UCP2/3—likely to be fundamental for mitochondrial Ca 2+ uniport. Nat Cell Biol, 2008; 10(11):1237–40.

Trumbeckaite S, Kuliaviene I, Deduchovas O, Kincius M, Baniene R, Virketyte S, Bukauskas D, Jansen E, Kupčinskas L, Borutaite V, Gulbinas A. Experimental acute pancreatitis induces mitochondrial dysfunction in rat pancreas, kidney and lungs but not in liver. Pancreatology, 2013; 13(3):216–24.

Uc A, Andersen DK, Bellin MD, Bruce JI, Drewes AM, Engelhardt JF, Forsmark CE, Lerch MM, Lowe ME, Neuschwander-Tetri BA, O'Keefe SJ. Chronic pancreatitis in the 21st century-research challenges and opportunities: summary of a National Institute of Diabetes and Digestive and Kidney Diseases Workshop. Pancreas, 2016; 45(10):1365.

Waldron RT, Su HY, Piplani H, Capri J, Cohn W, Whitelegge JP, Faull KF, Sakkiah S, Abrol R, Yang W, Zhou B. Ethanol induced disordering of pancreatic acinar cell endoplasmic reticulum: an ER stress/defective unfolded protein response model. Cell Mol Gastroenterol Hepatol, 2018; 5(4):479–97.

Weniger M, Reinelt L, Neumann J, Holdt L, Ilmer M, Renz B, Hartwig W, Werner J, Bazhin AV, D'Haese JG. The analgesic effect of the mitochondria-targeted antioxidant SkQ1 in pancreatic inflammation. Oxid Med Cell Longev, 2016; 2016:4650489.

Wu J, Luo X, Yan LJ. Two dimensional blue native/SDS-PAGE to identify mitochondrial complex I subunits modified by 4-hydroxynonenal (HNE). Front Physiol, 2015; 6:98.

Ye R, Mareninova OA, Barron E, Wang M, Hinton DR, Pandol SJ, Lee AS. Grp78 heterozygosity regulates chaperone balance in exocrine pancreas with differential response to cerulein-induced acute pancreatitis. Am J Pathol, 2010; 177(6):2827–36.

Zang Q, Maass DL, White J, Horton JW. Cardiac mitochondrial damage and loss of ROS defense after burn injury: the beneficial effects of antioxidant therapy. J Appl Physiol, 2007; 102(1):103–12.

Zeeshan H, Lee G, Kim HR, Chae HJ. Endoplasmic reticulum stress and associated ROS. Int J Mol Sci, 2016; 17(3):327.

Zhou R, Yazdi AS, Menu P, Tschopp J. A role for mitochondria in NLRP3 inflammasome activation. Nature, 2011; 469(7329):221–5.

How to cite this article:
Srikantam S, Arumugam G. Glycyrrhizin modulates ER stress-induced UPR and concomitant mitochondrial dysfunction and activation of NF-κB in alcohol and cerulein-induced pancreatitis in rats. J Appl Pharm Sci, 2021; 11(03):130–140.

6. SUMMARY

Chronic pancreatitis arises when the pancreas becomes injured by long-standing inflammation, mostly caused by alcohol abuse. Inflammation impairs pancreatic functions gradually with long-standing abdominal pain as the major clinical symptom. Poor functional pancreas causes improper digestion of fats, altered blood sugar levels, nutritional deficiencies and weight loss. If left unmonitored, CP can increase the risk of pancreatic cancer. Diagnosis is challenging in CP as symptoms are similar to that of ulcers, gallstones, irritable bowel syndrome, or even pancreatic cancer. Blood tests, which can detect the digestive enzyme leakage, out of the pancreas into the bloodstream, when the pancreas is inflamed are very reliable markers.

Traditional herbal medicine, which take advantage of the plant extracts, is dominating the treatment of chronic diseases in recent times. Here by, we focused one such traditional herb, *Glycyrrhiza glabra* and its major phytoconstituent glycyrrhizin against alcohol and cerulein-induced rat model of CP. The present study was aimed to give scientific evidence for the pancreato-protective effect of HAELR and GZ which are traditionally used for inflammation related disorders. Experimental rats were subjected to alcohol and cerulein induced inflammation and treated with the test drugs. HAELR and glycyrrhizin exhibited excellent pancreato-protective activity against various pathobiologies of CP and, the obtained results are summarized below:

- HAELR was subjected to GCMS analysis, and it revealed the presence of biologically important phytochemicals like 3-hydroxy-3,4,5,7-tetramethoxyflavone, jaceidin triacetate and undecane.

- HPLC-UV analysis conducted, revealed the presence of flavonoids like rutin, luteolin, thymoquinone and galangin at a concentration of 0.9 mg/g, 0.6 mg/g, 0.5 mg/g, and 1.3 mg/g, respectively and saponins like glycyrrhzin at a concentration of 0.02 mg/g in HAELR.

- The predicted oral rat LD_{50} for GZ was estimated by nearest neighbor method using TEST software tool. It was found to be 88.39 mg/kg body weight.

- The LD_{50} value of HAELR was found to be greater than 5000 mg/kg body weight.

- Acute toxicity study was carried out with the concentrations of 500, 1000, 2000, 4000 and 5000 mg/kg b.wt. of HAELR for 14days and sub-chronic toxicity study with concentrations of 50, 100, 200,400 and 500 mg/kg b.wt. for 90 days. No adverse effects were noted. No mortality was observed upto 5000mg/kg b. wt, highlighting the safety of HAELR. This was evidenced by biochemical, hematological and histopathological investigations besides various other general observations.

- There observed no notable changes in morphology, behavior or physiology during acute and chronic exposures of HAELR.And there observed no significant changes either in the body weight or relative organ weights.

- Acute and chronic exposures of HAELR did not cause any prominent alteration in the liver,heart and kidney functions as indicated by their respective biochemical markers. No drastic change was observed either in the oxidative status or hematological system, upon acute and chronic exposures of HAELR.

- The histopathological examinations were conducted on liver, kidney, heart, pancreas and brain tissues. Acute and chronic exposures of HAELR did not cause any abnormalities or tissue architecture alterations.

- Dose response studies were conducted with 25, 50, 100 and 200 mg/kg b.wt. of HAELR and 2.5, 5, 10 and 20 mg/kg b.wt. of GZ. The pancreatic markers like lipase and amylase, and inflammatory markers like MPO, caspase-1, IL-1 β and IL-18 were assessed. Both the markers were found elevated during EtOH and Cer-induced pancreatitis. HAELR/GZ co-administrations were observed to restore them. The doses of 100 mg/kg b.wt of HAELR and 10 mg/kg b.wt of

GZ, which exhibited maximum pancreato-protective effect against EtOH and Cer-induced pancreatitis, were selected for carrying out further investigations.

- The therapeutic efficacy of HAELR and GZ against EtOH and Cer-induced pancreatitis was investigated in detail and the results are: The pancreatitis marker enzymes like lipase and amylase activities were found elevated in serum significantly, upon administration of EtOH and Cer. HAELR/GZ co-administrations observed to have restored these levels significantly confirming their protectivity against pancreatic injury.

- Cellular oxidative stress was measured through total peroxide content, TAC and OSI; GSH, GPx, SOD and CAT activities. Lipid peroxidation was measured through determinations of TBARS and 4-HNE.Oxidative stress and lipid peroxidation were found elevated significantly during EtOH and Cer-induced pancreatitis. Whereas, HAELR/GZ co-administration found to ameliorate these pathological changes.

- Inflammation was measured through activity of pancreatic MPO, and serum levels of caspase-1, IL-1 β, and IL-18. It was found increased significantly during EtOH and Cer-induced pancreatitis. The levels of these inflammatory mediators were found restored with HAELR/GZ co-administrations indicating the attenuation of pancreatic inflammation by HAELR and GZ.

- mRNA expression of NF-κB was studied to monitor inflammation in pancreas. It was found elevated significantly during EtOH and Cer-induced pancreatitis, as evidenced from RT-PCR analysis. It was observed to be ameliorated with HAELR/GZ co-administrations.

- mRNA expression of the UPR genes (ATF4, GRP78, CHOP and XBP1) were studied to monitor ER stress in pancreas. They were found upregulated significantly indicating the chronically activated ER stress during EtOH and Cer-induced pancreatitis. HAELR/GZ co-administrations were observed to ameliorate the increased expression, underlining their role in protecting against pathologic ER stress in CP.

- Oxidative stress was assessed in pancreatic mitochondria. A significant decrease in GSH content, antioxidant enzymes (GPx, SOD, CAT) and a significant increase in lipid peroxidation products (TBARS,4-HNE) were observed in mitochondria during EtOH and Cer-induced pancreatitis, indicating association of CP with mitochondrial oxidative stress. HAELR/GZ co-administrations were recorded to enhance the anti-oxidative capacity of mitochondria as evidenced from the attenuated levels of antioxidants.

- The intra-mitochondrial free calcium levels were determined and were found increased significantly upon EtOH and Cer administration. This is due to the gradual release of Ca 2+ from ER under the influence of alcoholic metabolites like FAEEs. This increase was not observed with HAELR/GZ co-administrations emphasizing attenuation of [Ca 2+] m overload in mitochondria by HAELR/GZ.

- Mitochondrial functional alteration was monitored through complex-1 activity. Pronounced inhibition of complex-1 activity of mitochondrial respiratory chain was observed during EtOH and Cer-induced pancreatitis, pointing out the decline in energy formation. It was observed to be re-established upon HAELR/GZ co-administrations.

- Histopathological studies were conducted to add more evidence for the therapeutic efficacy of HAELR and GZ. It revealed the presence of prominent inflammation and fibrosis during EtOH and Cer-induced pancreatitis. These pathological alterations in pancreatic tissue architecture were found to be minimized by HAELR/GZ co-administration.

- The Spearman's rank correlation test was conducted between GRP78 vs 4-HNE; CHOP vs IL-1β, $[Ca^{2+}]_m$; $[Ca^{2+}]_m$ vs complex-1, TBARS and GSH; CHOP vs NF-κB. In this study, a correlated effect was observed between ER stress and mitochondrial dysfunction, the key mechanisms contributing to the pathobiology of CP as indicated by a positive correlation found between GRP78 vs 4-HNE and CHOP vs IL-1β, $[Ca^{2+}]_m$.

- An *insilico* molecular docking analysis was carried out to understand the effect of GZ on ER stress. The docking energy between GZ vs GRP78 and ATF4 was found to be -5.82 kcal/mol and -5.8 kcal/mol respectively. This analysis gives base level evidence for the binding affinity between GZ and the target proteins GRP78 and ATF4.This would be true and mimic, the affinity and interaction invivo.

7. CONCLUSION

Results of the current investigation has shown that, HAELR is rich in phytochemicals with a wide variety of pharmacological activities. HAELR/ glycyrrhizin plays a key role in decreasing the pathological modifications of alcohol and cerulein-induced pancreatitis. HAELR/glycyrrhizin exerts significant pancreato-protective properties, probably by mitigating the ER stress and its consequent mitochondrial dysfunction and oxidative stress, and there by the inflammation. In this regard, HAELR/GZ inhibits ER stress by downregulating its UPR components-ATF4, GRP78, CHOP and XBP1. Furthermore, HAELR/glycyrrhizin downregulates expression of NF-κB and its consequent maturation of pro-inflammatory cytokines, responsible for regulating the level of inflammation in pancreas. GZ was observed to have had a good binding affinity towards GRP78 and ATF4 in *insilico* molecular docking. Thus, HAELR/GZ can be considered as potent drugs for the treatment of pancreatitis which targets ER stress followed by mitochondrial dysfunction and NF-κB activation, resulting in the mitigation of maturation and release of pro-inflammatory cytokines in pancreas, offering protection to the organ.

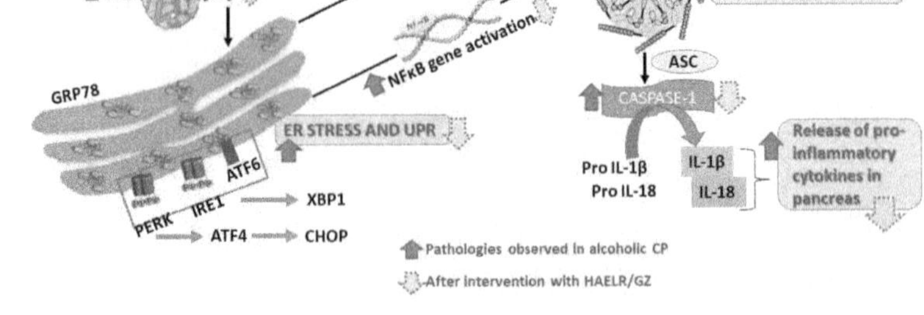

The tentative highlight on the mode of action of HAELR/GZ

8. FUTURE PROSPECTS OF THESTUDY

The study warrants the need to extrapolate the obtained results of this animal study, to clinical trials and check whether this kind of intervention with HAELR/GZ could reduce the disease severity of alcoholic CP in human beings also.

CPSIA information can be obtained
at www.ICGtesting.com
Printed in the USA
LVHW012115291122
734192LV00014B/544

9 781805 459897